Every Decker
book is
accompanied
by a CD-ROM.

The disc appears in the front of each copy, in its own
sealed jacket.

The disc contains the complete text and illustrations
of the book, in fully searchable PDF files. The book
and disc are sold *only* as a package; neither is available
indepe
items

BC D   ity
elec
info

We   ble
and

er
sher

*PDQ** SERIES

ACKERMANN
PDQ PHYSIOLOGY

BAKER, MURRAY
PDQ BIOCHEMISTRY

CORMACK
PDQ HISTOLOGY

INGLE
PDQ ENDODONTICS

JOHNSON
PDQ PHARMACOLOGY, 2/e

KERN
PDQ HEMATOLOGY

McKIBBON
PDQ EVIDENCE-BASED PRINCIPLES AND PRACTICE

NORMAN, STREINER
PDQ STATISTICS, 2/e

SCHLAGENHAUF, FUNK
PDQ TRAVELERS' MALARIA

SCIUBBA
PDQ ORAL DISEASE: DIAGNOSIS AND TREATMENT

STREINER, NORMAN
PDQ EPIDEMIOLOGY, 2/e

---

*PDQ (Pretty Darned Quick)

PDQ INTEGRATIVE ONCOLOGY
Complementary Therapies in Cancer Care

BARRIE R. CASSILETH, MS, PhD
Chief, Integrative Medicine Service
Memorial Sloan-Kettering Cancer Center
New York, New York

GARY DENG, MD, PhD
ANDREW VICKERS, PhD
K. SIMON YEUNG, RPh, LAc
Integrative Medicine Service
Memorial Sloan-Kettering Cancer Center
New York, New York

with contributions by
Marcin Chwistek, MD
Donald Garrity, RD, CDN
Jyothirmai Gubili, MS
Patricia Vroom, PhD

2005
BC Decker Inc
Hamilton • London

BC Decker Inc
P.O. Box 620, L.C.D. 1
Hamilton, Ontario L8N 3K7
Tel: 905-522-7017; 1-800-568-7281
Fax: 905-522-7839; 1-888-311-4987
E-mail: info@bcdecker.com
www.bcdecker.com

04 05 06 07/WPC/9 8 7 6 5 4 3 2 1

ISBN 1-55009-280-4

Printed in the United States of America

Sales and Distribution

United States
BC Decker Inc
P.O. Box 785
Lewiston, NY 14092-0785
Tel: 905-522-7017; 800-568-7281
Fax: 905-522-7839; 888-311-4987
E-mail: info@bcdecker.com
www.bcdecker.com

Canada
BC Decker Inc
20 Hughson Street South
P.O. Box 620, LCD 1
Hamilton, Ontario L8N 3K7
Tel: 905-522-7017; 800-568-7281
Fax: 905-522-7839; 888-311-4987
E-mail: info@bcdecker.com
www.bcdecker.com

Foreign Rights
John Scott & Company
International Publishers' Agency
P.O. Box 878
Kimberton, PA 19442
Tel: 610-827-1640
Fax: 610-827-1671
E-mail: jsco@voicenet.com

Japan
Igaku-Shoin Ltd.
Foreign Publications Department
3-24-17 Hongo
Bunkyo-ku, Tokyo
Japan 113-8719
Tel: 3 3817 5680
Fax: 3 3815 6776
E-mail: fd@igaku-shoin.co.jp

U.K., Europe, Scandinavia,
  Middle East
Elsevier Science
Customer Service Department
Foots Cray High Street
Sidcup, Kent
DA14 5HP, UK
Tel: 44 (0) 208 308 5760
Fax: 44 (0) 181 308 5702
E-mail: cservice@harcourt.com

Singapore, Malaysia,Thailand,
  Philippines, Indonesia,
  Vietnam, Pacific Rim, Korea
Elsevier Science Asia
583 Orchard Road
#09/01, Forum
Singapore 238884
Tel: 65-737-3593
Fax: 65-753-2145

Australia, New Zealand
Elsevier Science Australia
Customer Service Department
STM Division
Locked Bag 16
St. Peters, New South Wales, 2044
Australia
Tel: 61 02 9517-8999
Fax: 61 02 9517-2249
E-mail: stmp@harcourt.com.au
Web site: www.harcourt.com.au

Mexico and Central America
ETM SA de CV
Calle de Tula 59
Colonia Condesa
06140 Mexico DF, Mexico
Tel: 52-5-5553-6657
Fax: 52-5-5211-8468
E-mail: editoresdetextosmex@
  prodigy.net.mx

Brazil
Tecmedd
Av. Maurílio Biagi,, 2850
City Ribeirão Preto – SP – CEP:
  14021-000
Tel: 0800 992236
Fax: (16) 3993-9000

India, Bangladesh, Pakistan, Sri
  Lanka
Elsevier Health Sciences Division
Customer Service Department
17A/1, Main Ring Road
Lajpat Nagar IV
New Delhi – 110024, India
Tel: 91 11 2644 7160-64
Fax: 91 11 2644 7156
E-mail: esindia@vsnl.net

Preface

Patients, always our best teachers, awakened me to the importance of complementary modalities almost three decades ago—it became clear that many patients and family members were looking outside of mainstream practice for additional answers to the problems they faced. Many were also drawn to what were then called "questionable" or unproven methods, which remain in the form of non-viable, so-called "alternatives" to mainstream cancer treatment.

About this time, advances in chemotherapy, radiation, and surgery greatly increased the numbers of cancer patients successfully treated for their disease. But improvements in therapy came then, as now, with a price: Difficult physical and emotional side effects.

Patients sought broader and better supportive care for pain and other treatment sequelae, as well as additional means of maintaining their health in the form of we today call, "complementary therapies," interventions that mitigate symptoms, enhance quality of life, and possibly keep disease at bay.

Eventually the scientific community began to study the documentable benefits of these therapies, as governments and individual researchers developed interests in acupuncture, herbs and other botanicals, touch therapies, and so on. This manual is for oncology professionals in hope of advancing the field of Integrative Oncology, interesting others in the scientific investigation of complementary modalities and botanicals in oncology, and encouraging the application of useful therapies in cancer care.

We thank the patients and families who press for rightful attention to their needs and who continue to provide us with guidance and ideas. We join them, convinced that adjunctive complementary therapies help in non-invasive ways.

The senior authors also thank Marcin Chwistek, Donald Garrity, Jyothirmai Gubili, and Pat Vroom for contributing to chapters in this manual. Jyothi Gubili also helped with editing and in many other ways. Without Carolyn Nicholson and Joanne Fraser's administrative and office support, little could have been accomplished. We very much appreciate Brian Decker's encouragement and support of this venture.

BRC

May, 2005

This book is dedicated to the memory of Laurance S. Rockefeller, whose vision sought to improve the care and well being of those afflicted with cancer.

Contents

SECTION I: Source and Practice   **1**
of Complementary Therapies

1. Introduction (Terminology and Regulatory Issues) 3
2. Other Medical Paradigms 8
3. Herbs and Other Botanicals .17
4. Botanicals, Cancer and Herb-Drug Interactions 33
5. Diet and Nutrition 42
6. Vitamins and Dietary Supplements 52
7. Mind-Body Therapies 65
8. Acupuncture 73
9. Bodywork 82
10. Using the Senses 87

SECTION II: Complementary Therapies   **93**
by Cancer Diagnosis

11. Breast Cancer 95
12. Gastrointestinal Cancers 106
13. Lung Cancer 115
14. Prostate Cancer 123

SECTION III: Complementary Therapies   **133**
by the Symptoms They Treat

15. Pain 135
16. Mood Disturbance and Fatigue 145
17. Gastrointestinal Symptoms 157
18. Endocrine Symptoms 167
19. Alternative/Questionable Therapies 172

INDEX   **178**

Part I

SOURCE AND PRACTICE OF COMPLEMENTARY THERAPIES

Introduction to Integrative Oncology

Integrative oncology, the synthesis of mainstream cancer treatment and effective complementary therapies, expands a long tradition of supportive care in oncology. The profound public and cancer patient interest in complementary modalities arose in the context of new emphases on quality of life in oncology research and treatment, patients' desire to play a role in regaining and maintaining their health, imperfect mainstream interventions for symptom relief, the attraction to the individualized comfort of complementary therapies in increasingly brief and impersonal medical care, in addition to doubtless many other trends.

The very mysticism of the ancient healing traditions that gird many complementary modalities is itself appealing, perhaps because it ties us to enduring, prescientific traditions that have provided comfort and solace since the beginning of history. A large majority of patients with cancer seek modern oncologic treatment, not complementary or alternative therapies, to treat their disease. They also want the many benefits that adjunctive complementary therapies provide, especially those that effectively control symptoms with comforting, noninvasive techniques. Those techniques are reviewed throughout this manual.

PREVALENCE

Complementary and alternative medicine (CAM) is markedly prevalent among cancer patients. A systematic review of 26 surveys of cancer patients conducted in 13 countries found an average prevalence of 31%, with rates ranging up to 64%. Subsequent studies report even broader prevalence—up to 83%—depending on definitions of CAM applied. The 2002 Datamonitor Survey covering the

United States and Europe indicates that 80% of cancer patients use alternative or complementary modalities.

Virtually all studies conducted internationally of both cancer patients and the general public indicate that those who seek CAM therapies are better educated, of higher socioeconomic status, female, and younger than those who do not. Typically, they are more health conscious and use more mainstream medical services than do others. Most studies find that patients use CAM primarily for three reasons: because they want to improve physiologic and psychosocial well-being; because they value the closer relationships possible with CAM practitioners; and because they want more control over and greater responsibility for self-care.

Increasing interest in complementary therapies among patients has been matched by mounting scientific attention and the development of research and clinical programs in integrative medicine at major cancer centers, including Memorial Sloan-Kettering, M. D. Anderson, Dana-Farber, University of California at San Francisco, and many others. The quality of research has advanced accordingly, and now an increasing folio of solid data enables confident clinical recommendations for a reasonable number of approaches.

THE EVOLVING TERMINOLOGY OF CAM

CAM is a general term used to describe a broad range of disparate, largely unrelated techniques. The convenient acronym actually provides a disservice. It inappropriately links unrelated interventions, including unproven or disproved "alternatives" that are helpful to no one, and adjunctive "complementary" therapies that are evidence-based and quite helpful to most. Oxygen healing, iridology, and colonic irrigation, dubious cancer therapies all, do not belong under the same umbrella term with yoga, meditation, and music therapy. Rather, these form two distinct categories.

We have long promoted what we view as a necessary distinction between complementary and alternative therapies. Complementary therapies are used as adjuncts to mainstream cancer care. They are supportive measures that control symptoms, enhance well-being, and contribute to overall patient care. Alternative therapies, conversely, typically are promoted for use instead of mainstream treatment. Interventions sold as literal alternatives to chemotherapy, surgery, and radiation therapy tend to be biologically active, extremely costly, and potentially harmful, especially when they delay needed care. This is especially problematic in oncology, since delayed treatment can diminish the possibility of remission or cure.

A small minority of patients is drawn to promotional claims for "more natural" alternatives to surgery, chemotherapy, and radiation therapy. Imperfect though they may be, these are the best treatments available today, and with technology for screening and early detection, they are responsible for the higher than 60% cure rate across cancer diagnoses in the United States. In underdeveloped countries such as India and China, where access to these advances is limited, the overall cancer cure rate remains at about 20%.

The higher cure rates produce larger numbers of cancer survivors—approximately 10 million in the United States today, according to the American Cancer Society. It also grants us the good fortune to address not only tumor destruction in oncology, but also the important issues of patient and survivor quality of life. This is where complementary therapies play a significant role. As they are proven safe and effective, these therapies become part of mainstream care, producing integrative oncology, a synthesis of the best of mainstream treatment and rational, data-based, adjunctive techniques.

Such integration is evolving. The terms "integrative medicine" or "integrative oncology" are now applied to programs in North America, the United Kingdom, Europe, and elsewhere. Further, an international Society for Integrative Oncology—the first such organization—was formed recently by leading oncologists and cancer centers to encourage high-quality scientific research and appropriate application of complementary modalities.

These are indicators not only of the necessary semantic shift, but also of complementary modality assimilation into mainstream cancer research and care. Complementary therapies can either be passive, such as massage therapy and acupuncture, or require active patient involvement, such as self-hypnosis, yoga, and meditation. Some patients prefer passive interventions, some favor active participation, and many use both, depending on the problem they hope to address. A majority, however, appreciate the opportunity to contribute to their own care. In addition to their clinical utility, complementary therapies enable patients to select and participate in their cancer treatment. These are highly valued and significant opportunities.

One area of active patient engagement is that of dietary supplements. Concerns arise here because no government agency assures the safety and efficacy of these readily available products, which include herbs and other botanicals, unusual and high-dose vitamin or mineral preparations, and a wide variety of other nonprescription remedies. Virtually anyone may create an agent, put it in a bottle, and place the bottle on health food store shelves. The North American market is $17.7 billion annually, according to MarketResearch.com. This is a special issue in cancer patient care, because many dietary supplements may interfere or interact negatively with chemotherapeutic agents and other prescription pharmaceuticals. Supplements also may be contaminated or produce undesirable side effects (see Chapter 4).

The hands-off government policy resulted from a major, multimillion dollar lobbying effort on the part of the dietary supplement industry, which urged Americans to "Write to Congress today, or kiss your supplements good-bye!" This false message resulted in passage of the 1994 Dietary Supplement and Health Education Act, which created a protective new category for the approximately 20,000 vitamins, minerals, herbs, and all else that had been sold as a supplement prior to October 1994.

This means that supplements are protected from government scrutiny. The US Food and Drug Administration (FDA) may halt production of a product not because the manufacturer fails to show it is safe and effective—manufacturers are not so required—but after the FDA itself provides proof that the agent may be dangerous. Manufacturers must indicate that a product is not intended to diagnose, treat, cure, or prevent any disease, but they are permitted to describe how the product can affect the consumer's structure, function, or general well-being. As cases of adverse effects have surfaced during recent years, an increase has occurred in efforts to tighten regulations of the sale and use of supplements.

Following discussion of the source and practice of complementary therapies, this manual summarizes therapies by major cancer diagnoses and concludes with a section on the management of major symptoms. A final chapter reviews currently popular but questionable alternative therapies. Our hope is that this information will facilitate dialogue with patients and help broaden the approach to cancer treatment that integrative oncology can engender. Come join us in this promising new endeavor.

READINGS AND RESOURCES

1. Adams J, Sibbritt DW, Easthope G, et al. The profile of women who consult alternative health practitioners in Australia. Med J Aust 2003;179:297–300.
2. Cassileth BR, Deng G. Complementary and alternative therapies in cancer. Oncologist 2004;9:80–9.
3. Datamonitor. Complementary and alternative medicines in cancer therapy. Publication BFHC0462. Available at http://www.datamonitor.com/all/reports/product_summary.asp?pid=BFHC0462 (accessed February 11, 2005).
4. Jemal A, Clegg LX, Ward E, et al. Annual report to the nation on the status of cancer, 1975–2001, with a special feature regarding survival. Cancer 2004;101:3–27.
5 Society for Integrative Oncology. http://www.integrativeonc.org (accessed February 11, 2005).

2

Other Medical Paradigms

Healing systems from ancient cultures are of interest not only for historical reasons, but also for what they can teach us today. Some aspects of these approaches, such as meditation and yoga from Ayurveda and acupuncture from traditional Chinese medicine (TCM), have been scientifically studied and shown to have substantial contemporary benefit (see Chapters 7 and 8). These medical systems, as well as homeopathy and naturopathy, are described in this chapter as examples of medical paradigms that preceded current scientific understanding of human physiology and disease. They exist today essentially as originally conceived, in contrast to Western medicine, which constantly changes as new information clarifies understanding of health and illness and as research leads to new therapeutic interventions.

AYURVEDA

The origins of Ayurveda go back to 1500 BC, when Aryans from central Asia invaded India, bringing with them their "Vedas" (Sanskrit for "knowledge") comprised of literature, hymns, teachings, manuscripts, and prayers. Vedas formed the basis of India's moral, religious, and cultural codes, as well as its medical system. Ayurvedic ("knowledge of life") medicine, expanded over time, is still practiced by many in India.

Basic Concepts

The basic premise of Ayurveda is that the body, mind, and spirit are intimately connected, a belief not unlike that understood today. A separation of mind and spirit from the body results in physical imbalance and disease. Restoring this harmony will return the individual to health and well being. This concept and many other Ayurvedic principles are similar to those of TCM. Both systems are based on concepts of life force and the vital relationship among body, mind, and nature, and on restoring good health through exercise, proper diet, and meditation. Both rely on tongue and pulse examination for diagnostic purposes.

According to Ayurvedic principles, every individual has a unique constitution and formula for good health. The maintenance of inward balance and harmony with the environment and nature requires diet and exercise unique to each individual's constitution, or *Prakruti*, which is a combination of the three principles (*doshas*) called Vata, Pitta, and Kapha. These are manifestations of the five basic elements: ether, air, fire, water, and earth. Vata (motion) constitution is a combination of ether and air; Pitta (metabolism) of fire and water; and Kapha (cohesiveness) earth and water.

Each basic element corresponds to one of the five senses: ether is related to hearing, air to touch, fire to sight, water to taste, and earth to smell. Color, emotions, seasons, and time of day also are interrelated (Figure 2-1).

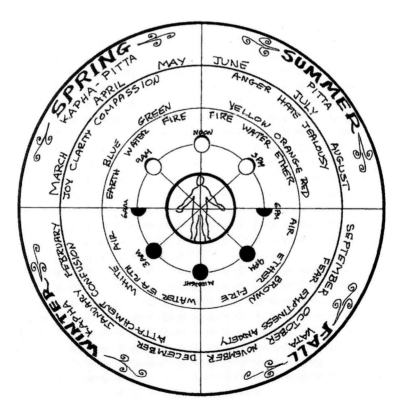

Figure 2-1 Ayurveda conceptualizes the interdependent relationship among all things in the cosmos.

Although each person is a combination of characteristics from all three doshas, a single dosha predominates, and it both determines and reflects one's physical, metabolic, and emotional characteristics, habits, and lifestyle.

Harmony among the doshas leads to good health. Imbalance—deficiency or excess—manifests itself as a symptom of disease. Maintaining and restoring health requires balancing the doshas, which is accomplished by reducing emotional stress, improving diet and lifestyle, and ridding the body of accumulated toxins. Diet and therapy are prescribed on the basis of the individual's predominant dosha type.

Life force, or *Prana* (equivalent to Chinese "Qi"), another important concept of Ayurveda, is believed to permeate all body organs and tissues. It is concentrated at various points along the midline of the body known as "chakras," which are believed to be linked to internal organs, natural elements, colors, and deities. Self-illumination is said to occur when energy reaches the topmost chakra.

Treatment

Diagnoses are described in terms of organ system disharmony or imbalance among doshas. The goal of treatment is to restore balance and harmony. Therapies are based on the individual's body type and include dietary and lifestyle recommendations, breathing exercises, and yoga. Herbs, spices, metals, and other natural product medicinals are prescribed. Removing toxins from the body, or *Panchakarma*, includes induced vomiting, enemas, bowel purgation, nasal administration of herbalized oils, and bloodletting.

Benefits and Cautions

Although many practitioners and followers of Ayurveda believe that regimens based on doshas can diagnose and treat all disorders, including serious illness, Ayurvedic healing techniques should not replace mainstream medical care for cancer or other illnesses. Some research documents the medicinal properties of Ayurvedic herbs such as turmeric, but the deliberate inclusion of heavy metals in herbal compounds for their assumed benefit, as in TCM, is of concern. In 2004, the US Centers for Disease Control and Prevention reported 12 cases of lead poisoning associated with the use of Ayurvedic medications.

Meditation, an essential component of ancient and contemporary Ayurvedic medicine, has been shown to reduce anxiety, help lower hypertension, and enhance general well-being (see Chapter 7). In the last few decades, however, a commercial trademarked version, "Transcendental Meditation," has emerged to the concern of many. Often described as a cult, it also promises its followers unlikely abilities such as flying, controlling the weather, and conquering aging. While meditation is an important component of Ayurvedic culture, "Transcendental Meditation," to the contrary, is a commercial enterprise that authorities believe draws young people into a private and exploitative world of potential harm.

TRADITIONAL CHINESE MEDICINE

TCM is a complete system of health in use for almost three millennia. The early medical text *Huang Di Nei Jing* ("The Yellow Emperor's Inner Classic") was compiled during the Han dynasty (206 BC–220 AD) It lists the medical knowledge accumulated during previous centuries of experience, and its principles are still applied today.

Basic Concepts

The cornerstone concept in TCM is *Qi*, generally described as energy flow. It is believed that pain and symptoms of disease occur when the flow of Qi is impaired. Another governing principle is yin–yang, the Taoist concept of balance, which holds that everything has an equal but opposite counterpart in nature. For example, night–day, female–male, and right–left components are opposing, yet they complement each other's existence (Table 2-1). As in ancient Ayurveda, TCM includes the belief that the human body exists in harmony when all yin–yang factors coexist in balance and that disharmony causes disease. Healing requires restoring that balance.

The ancient Chinese used the relationships seen in nature to explain disease states. Descriptions of human anatomy often reflect the surrounding landscape, and organ function is assigned to five elements: wood, fire, earth, metal, and water. Similar to Ayurvedic understanding, the five elements in TCM are thought to mutually balance one another in a harmonious cycle. Table 2-2 shows the interrelationships among the elements, the human body and mind, and the seasons.

Table 2-1

YIN AND YANG COMPONENTS

Yang	Yin
Light	Dark
Day	Night
Hot	Cold
Male	Female
External	Internal

Table 2-2

THE FIVE ELEMENT CORRESPONDENCES

Category	Wood	Fire	Earth	Metal	Water
Viscus	Liver	Heart	Spleen	Lungs	Kidney
Bowel	Gallbladder	Small intestine	Stomach	Large intestine	Urinary bladder
Season	Spring	Summer	Transition	Autumn	Winter
Taste	Sour	Bitter	Sweet	Pungent	Salty
Sense organ	Eyes	Tongue	Mouth	Nose	Ears
Emotion	Anger	Joy	Thought	Sorrow	Fear

Treatment

Patients are treated with herbal compounds consisting of up to 20 different botanical, mineral, or animal products (see Chapters 3 and 4), dietary modification, and acupuncture (see Chapter 8) to correct the improper flow of Qi. Qigong and tai chi are breathing, exercise, and meditation techniques also prescribed to balance and strengthen Qi and to maintain health (see Chapter 7).

Some components of TCM have been documented by modern research as effective. Camptothecan, a chemotherapeutic agent, was derived from a Chinese herb. Major clinical trials indicate that acupuncture is effective against chronic pain, chemotherapy-related nausea, and other symptoms associated with cancer and cancer treatment (see Chapter 8). Qigong enhances pulmonary function and is especially useful for the elderly or patients with cancer; meditation and massage lower anxiety and increase feelings of relaxation; tai chi effectively improves balance and muscle tone in the elderly (see Chapters 7 and 9).

Benefits and Cautions

Many aspects of TCM enhance well-being and have other important roles in health care. Herbal remedies are biologically active and can produce adverse effects if used inappropriately (improper use of ephedra has caused fatalities). Some herbs are hepatotoxic, and many are not appropriate for patients under treatment for cancer (see Chapter 4). Standards to maintain quality control in the development and processing of botanical agents are lacking and needed.

HOMEOPATHY

Homeopathy is briefly reviewed here to provide an understanding of this method, as some cancer patients may ask about it. An approach developed by German physician Samuel Hahnemann 200 years ago, homeopathy remains popular especially in European countries but also has adherents in North America. The word homeopathy derives from the Greek words *homoios* (similar) and *pathos* (suffering). Homeopathic products typically contain not even one molecule of the active ingredient and are promoted as safe alternatives to harsher treatments.

Basic Concepts

The practice of homeopathy is governed by the Law of Similars, "like cures like." Hahnemann and his followers concluded that while certain products cause specific symptoms when ingested by healthy individuals, a highly diluted form of the same substance could relieve similar symptoms in patients. The dilution process involves adding a small amount of a plant, animal, or mineral to distilled water or another substrate, shaking vigorously, then repeating the dilution and shaking process up to 30,000 times. The dilution and shaking process is said to "increase the potency of the medicine." When asked how a product can act against disease when it does not contain even one molecule of the original substance, homeopaths explain that the product retains a "memory" of the original substance.

Treatment

Patients provide lengthy details about their life (it has been noted that the interview process itself may be a healing experience), and physical examination and laboratory tests are conducted as needed for diagnosis. Treatment involves use of a designated highly diluted ("homeopathic") preparation. Preparations that are even further diluted are used to treat chronic disease.

Benefits and Cautions

The majority of patients seek homeopathic attention to treat chronic and transient conditions such as arthritis, asthma, colds, flu, and allergies. Although some practitioners believe that their homeopathic remedies can cure any illness, these remedies are no substitute for insulin in diabetes or medical treatment, for cancer or any acute or serious disease. Homeopathic remedies are free of toxicity and side effects. The only danger lies in patients who use them thereby postponing mainstream care for serious illness or injury. While homeopathic remedies cannot hurt self-limiting ailments, no published evidence indicates a role for homeopathy in cancer treatment. Most scientists suggest that homeopathic remedies provide a placebo response, as homeopathic concepts and treatment contradict modern scientific understanding.

NATUROPATHY

Naturopathy, the youngest alternative medical paradigm noted here, originated toward the end of the nineteenth century. Unlike systems that developed well before modern understanding of human physiology and disease, naturopathy shares current understanding of anatomy and physiology and uses mainstream diagnostic techniques.

Basic Concepts

Naturopathy aims to assist nature and to facilitate the body's inherent healing mechanisms. In the 1900s, Benedict Lust brought naturopathy to the United States and advocated for its adoption. He was strongly opposed to vaccination because it refuted the naturopathic view that people, not microorganisms, bring disease upon themselves. Some naturopaths still maintain that early belief.

Naturopathic doctors (NDs) are trained in four-year postgraduate programs. The first two years include courses in biochemistry and anatomy, the second two years consist of course work in herbal medicine, homeopathy, and, often, acupuncture. A residency with an experienced naturopath may follow, to learn treating the whole person and understanding overall lifestyle, environment, and interactions that influence well-being, but ND graduates may elect to go directly into practice.

Treatment

Nutrition and lifestyle measures that coincide with current government recommendations, homeopathic remedies, and treatment with botanicals and plants are primary. Naturopathy emphasizes preventive care, including healthful diets and lifestyles, to ward off the development of disease. Naturopaths also perform minor surgical procedures. Typical naturopathic treatments are listed in Table 2-3.

Benefits and Cautions

Naturopaths treat a wide range of illnesses from self-limiting, minor conditions to life-threatening diseases such as acquired immunodeficiency syndrome (AIDS) and cancer. Proponents view naturopathic medicine as an alternative to mainstream primary care, one that applies natural therapies with little toxicity. Naturopaths may refer patients to medical specialists when they perceive the need. Although

Table 2-3
NATUROPATHIC TREATMENTS

Therapeutic nutrition

Homeopathy
Plant substances
Manipulation of muscles, bone, and spine
Natural childbirth
Pre- and postnatal care
Acupuncture and other traditional Chinese medicine techniques
Counseling
Hypnotherapy
Hydrotherapy
Minor surgery

naturopathy may assist in treating minor health problems, it is not a viable substitute for medical care of major illness.

READINGS AND RESOURCES

1. American Cancer Society. http://www.cancer.org (accessed March 8, 2005).
2. Cassileth BR. The alternative medicine handbook: the complete reference guide to alternative and complementary therapies. New York: WW Norton; 1998.
3. National Center for Complementary and Alternative Medicines. National Institutes of Health. http://nccam.nih.gov/ (accessed March 8, 2005).
4. Quackwatch. http://www.quackwatch.org (accessed March 8, 2005).

3

Herbs and Other Botanicals

DEVELOPMENT OF BOTANICAL USE, STUDY, AND NOMENCLATURE

Since the dawn of human civilization, every culture on earth has used plants as medicine. Traditional medicine systems, including Native American healing, Indian Ayurveda, and traditional Chinese medicine (TCM), all incorporate botanicals in their therapeutic approaches. The ancient Chinese relied on natural substances, including those derived from plants, animals, and minerals, to treat disease. The first classic *Materia Medica*, compiled two thousand years ago during the rule of the Han dynasty, lists the applications and properties of 364 medicinal products, 70% of which are botanicals. Many are still in use today.

The World Health Organization estimates that 80% of the world's population uses plants as medicine today. In China, herbal medicines account for 30 to 50% of all medicine consumed. Up to 20 different herbs may be combined to create a formula for an individual based on that patient's current disease pattern. In the United States, over-the-counter herbal supplements have been increasingly popular in the last three decades. A double-digit percentage increase in herb sales occurred in the 1990s, and sales have remained at that level ever since.

According to the latest survey conducted by the Centers for Disease Control and Prevention, 19% of adults in the United States consumed botanicals in the past 12 months. Echinacea, ginseng, *Ginkgo biloba*, and garlic were the most commonly purchased. Cancer patients often use botanicals, typically in the belief that botanicals have fewer side effects than do conventional drugs. For example, a recent study in the

San Francisco Bay area revealed that over one-half of ovarian cancer patients surveyed used herbs following their diagnosis.

Most patients use herbs as an adjunctive treatment with chemotherapy or for palliation of symptoms without professional guidance. While herbal supplements are generally perceived as harmless, many reports in the literature indicate that misuse of these products can be detrimental. It is prudent for health care professionals to understand the properties and adverse effects of botanicals to provide much-needed advice to patients.

Although contemporary medicines are predominantly synthetic, many drugs, especially anticancer agents, are derived from botanicals. Also termed phytomedicinals, they are substances derived from plants, although algae, mushrooms, and other edible fungi also fall into this category. Phytomedicinals may contain the whole plant or its leaves, flowers, fruits, seeds, stem, wood, bark, roots, rhizomes, or exudates. The plant's fresh juices, gums, fixed oils, essential oils, resins, and dry powders also are used. Often two or more botanicals are combined to increase potency or produce fewer side effects. Excipients may be added to stabilize active components or enhance the overall effect. Final products take the form of powder, liquid, pills, or external preparations.

The study of botanicals as medicine ("herbalism") is called "herbology" when research concerns traditional theories and use of plants and their extracts. "Pharmacognosy," formed from the Greek words *pharmakon* (drug) and *gnosis* (knowledge), is a field covering information on medicine from natural sources, including animals and microorganisms as well as plants. The study of pharmacognosy was mandated in all pharmacy curricula in the United States until the 1980s. Since then, the teaching of natural products has been incorporated into other more general courses. Botanicals remain a focus of study in schools of naturopathy and traditional medicine.

Early classification efforts involved the appearance of plants. Through experience and observation, herbalists in both Eastern and Western civilizations came to believe that plants carry external clues to their medicinal properties. This is commonly known as the "Doctrine of Signatures." For example, because the root of ginseng resembles the human form, it is valued as a cure-all for human ailments. Similarly, the yellow goldenseal represents jaundice, and is therefore used to treat liver disease. Walnut has the shape of the brain or the kidney and is employed against symptoms related to these organs. Red-colored or heart-shaped leaves are often used to treat anemia or heart problems. Although the Doctrine of Signatures lacks a scientific basis, some of these effects have been verified by modern research.

Botanicals are known by their Latin, pharmaceutical, and common names (Table 3-1). They are given a generic (genus) and a specific (species) name according to the Latin binomial system of nomenclature. *Panax ginseng*, for example, holds the genus name *Panax* (from the Greek for "panacea") and the species name *ginseng*.

In many pharmaceutical references, botanicals are named according to "part of the plant used" followed by the scientific name. Radix ginseng ("radix" means "root") is an example.

Botanicals also are known by their common or native names. For example, ginseng is also termed *Ren Shen* (literally "human root" in Chinese).

Table 3-1

EXAMPLES OF BOTANICAL NOMENCLATURE

Latin Part Name	English Part Name	Pharmaceutical Name	Latin Binomial	Common Name
Cortex	Bark	Cortex cinnamomi	*Cinnamomum cassia*	Cinnamon bark
Flos	Flower	Flos lonicerae Japonicae	*Lonicera japonica*	Honeysuckle flower
Folium	Leaf	Folium ginkgo	*Ginkgo biloba*	Ginkgo leaf
Fructus	Fruit	Fructus crataegi	*Crataegus pinnatifida*	Hawthorn berry
Radix	Root	Radix ginseng	*Panax ginseng*	Ren Shen
Rhizoma	Underground stem	Rhizoma zingiberis	*Zingiber officinale*	Ginger root
Semen	Seed	Semen phaseoli radiati	*Phaseolus radiatus*	Mung bean

COLLECTION AND PROCESSING

Botanicals may be collected from their natural habitats or cultivated in farms or gardens. Herbs collected in the wild are believed to possess higher potency. This practice, however, is not encouraged. It is harmful to the ecosystem, and many plants have been driven to extinction by over-harvesting. In addition, misidentification of plant species and contamination of plants collected from polluted areas leading to toxicity have been reported. Today herbs are cultivated commercially in good agricultural practice (GAP) farms. These products tend to have a more consistent quality and predictable properties.

As natural products, the quality and properties of botanicals depend on the concentration of active components, which can be affected by the several factors. Climate and location, including soil conditions, rainfall and moisture, amount of daylight, fertilization, and other agricultural conditions, all affect the quality of botanicals harvested and the amount of active constituents they contain. For example, because of differences in climate, Indian cannabis yields 20% resin as compared with cannabis grown in Wisconsin, which yields only 6%.

Different parts of the plant also may contain varying concentrations of active components. For example, tetrahydrocannabinol (THC) is derived mainly from the resin concentrated in the leaves of the female cannabis plant. The seeds, however, have high concentrations of fixed oil, and the denatured form is used as a laxative in Chinese medicine. Time of harvest also influences the product. Herbs are collected when their active components are most abundant. In general, roots or rhizomes are harvested from immature plants, while branches, leaves, or the entire plant is collected during summer and autumn. Fruits and seeds usually are harvested when ripe. The bark of a plant usually is gathered in spring, when sap is most abundant.

Following harvesting, botanicals are sold as is or made into many types of products. Trained herbalists custom-formulate botanical remedies to each individual's unique condition, developing preparations from a single herb or from a combination. Some of these compounds are available at health food stores. Below are examples of the various forms that botanicals can take:

- The whole or part of the plant. These can be consumed directly as medicine or food. The herb or plant also may be processed by drying, fermenting, or cooking.

- Decoction. It is typically prepared with water as water is the most readily available solvent. Because heating increases the dissolution rate of soluble components, boiling or steeping herbs in hot water is the most common preparation method, and most herbs are consumed as tea or decoction.
- Extraction. Hydrophobic components are extracted from plants using alcohol as a solvent. The end product is called a tincture. Medicinal wines also are popular in traditional medicine.
- Powders or granules. Raw botanicals can be ground to powder for ease of dose titration and consumption. Often, solutes extracted from water or alcohol are dried into powder or granules to increase their potency and facilitate storage.
- Tablets and capsules. Traditionally, herbs are rolled manually into pills. Modern pharmaceutical practices have streamlined the production and preservation of herbs by encapsulating or pressing them to form coated tablets. This masks any disagreeable taste or odor and prolongs shelf life.
- External preparations. Botanicals have been formulated into salves, pastes, ointments, creams, balms, and lotions for external use to treat dermatologic problems and external trauma and for cosmetic products.
- Essential oils. The aroma of plants, especially from flowers, has long been recognized for its therapeutic properties. Volatile oils are extracted from many herbs for inhalation or to be used as perfume.

RESEARCH ON BOTANICALS AND CANCER

Many in vitro and animal studies have been conducted to determine the effects of various botanicals, but data from well-designed human clinical trials are limited. This could be because of the many challenges associated with botanicals research.

First, it is difficult to secure a patent for a natural substance. Pharmaceutical companies that spend the most money to support research are reluctant to invest funds and resources on products that do not ensure substantial financial return. Second, unlike synthetic pharmaceuticals, where a standard drug and dose regimen can be used for all patients, herbalists usually customize botanicals based on the individual's condition. This approach makes it difficult to

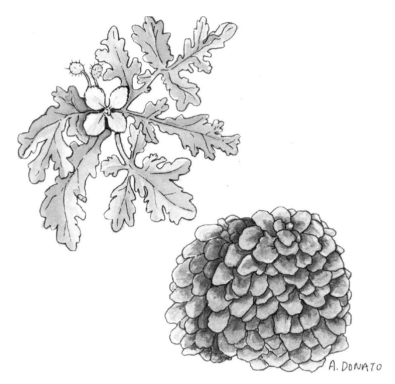

Figure 3-1 Huanglian, an herb, and Maitake, a mushroom extract, are under study in clinical trials for possible anticancer effects.

establish a dose range and study the interactions. Third, the properties of botanicals may vary between batches, complicating standardization and the study of biological effects. It is also difficult to obtain FDA approval for use of a variety of formulations in a single study.

However, the use of botanicals, especially Chinese herbs, is on the rise and research interest has strengthened accordingly. Some traditional formulas such as *Shi-quan-da-bu-tang* (or *Juzen-taiho-to* in Japanese) and *Xiao-chai-hu-tang* (*Sho-saiko-to* in Japanese) and modified formulas such as PC SPES appear to have anticancer effects and are under study in clinical trials. Individual botanicals such as Huang Lian and artemisia and phytochemicals such as indirubin and berberine show promising effects against cancers through different mechanisms of action. Examples of popular products with purported activity against cancer are given in Table 3-2.

Table 3-2

COMMONLY USED AGENTS WITH PURPORTED ANTICANCER PROPERTIES

Common Name	Mechanism of Action
Amygdalin	A naturally occurring cyanogenetic glycoside derived from nuts, plants, and the pits of certain fruits, primarily apricots. Although patients use amygdalin, commonly called Laetrile or vitamin B_{17}, research has demonstrated absence of beneficial effect. In 1982, a clinical trial involving 178 patients indicated that amygdalin is ineffective in treating cancer. Amygdalin is metabolized by beta-glucosidase to cyanide, benzaldehyde, and prunasin. Oral administration results in cyanide toxicity and death.
Nerium oleander	A hot water extract prepared from the aerial leaves of the *Nerium oleander* plant. The plant contains cardiac glycosides, primarily oleandrin, which is similar to digitalis. Raw leaves from the plant are toxic. In vitro studies indicate that Anvirzel, a commercial form of oleandrin, causes apoptosis in various cancer cell lines. One in vitro study showed that oleandrin increases the sensitivity of PC-3 human prostate cells to radiotherapy, but no animal or human data are available.
Astragalus	This is a common botanical used in TCM. The root contains polysaccharides that potentiate the immune-mediated antitumor activity of interleukin-2 in vitro. It also enhances the natural killer cell activity of normal subjects and potentiates activity of monocytes. The saponins of Astragalus root activate natural killer cells and increase phagocytosis. Studies done in China suggest that Astragalus, when used with angelica, exhibits renal protective effects by mediating gene expression. In vitro and animal, and anecdotal human data show Astragalus can reduce immunosuppression following chemotherapy. Although no significant adverse events have been reported related to Astragalus, patients on immunosuppressants (eg, tacrolimus or cyclosporin) should use this supplement with caution.

Table 3-2
CONTINUED

Common Name	Mechanism of Action
Artemisia	The plant is traditionally used for reducing fevers, inflammation, headache, and bleeding. It also has antimicrobial properties and has been used to treat malaria. Artemisinin, a compound derived from leaves, has been used to treat cancer in Asia. Studies have shown this compound to have antiproliferative, chemo-preventive, cytotoxic, and oncolytic effects on carcinoma cells. Artesunate, a semisynthetic derivative of artemisinin, has been shown to have an antiproliferative effect on medullary thyroid carcinoma cells. Eupatilin, a flavone extracted from *Artemisia asiatica*, has been shown to have cytotoxic effects on human promyelocytic leukemia cells.
Coriolus versicolor	This is an aqueous extract of the fruiting body and mycelium of the mushroom *Coriolus versicolor*. Patients use *Coriolus versicolor* or its constituents, polysaccharide-K (PSK) and polysaccharide-P (PSP) to stimulate the immune system, reduce chemotherapy toxicity, and increase the effectiveness of chemotherapy or radiotherapy for cancer. The glucans PSK and PSP show antiproliferative activity in animal models and immunostimulant activity in both animal and human studies. When used in conjunction with chemotherapy, PSK appears to improve survival rates in gastric and colorectal cancer patients after surgery. Outcomes in breast cancer, hepatocellular carcinoma, and leukemia are less impressive.
D-Limonene	Derived from the peels of citrus fruits. Patients use this supplement to prevent and treat cancer. D-Limonene is a cyclic monoterpene that causes G1 cell cycle arrest, induces apoptosis, and inhibits posttranslational modification of signal transduction proteins. In vitro and animal data suggest potential efficacy of D-limonene in treating cancer, but human data are lacking. Further research is necessary to determine if D-limonene has a role in the prevention or treatment of cancer.

Table 3-2
CONTINUED

Common Name	Mechanism of Action
Dong Guai	Derived from the root of the plant. Traditionally used for menstrual symptoms and as a female "tonic." Primary active ingredients include psoralens and safrole, both of which are thought to be carcinogenic. To date, clinical data regarding the use of Dong Quai for its proposed claims are inconclusive. Reported adverse events include diarrhea, photosensitivity, and gynecomastia. Due to its coumarin content, Dong Guai may interact with anticoagulant therapy.
Ellagic acid	A phenolic compound derived from red raspberries, strawberries, and walnuts. Ellagic acid has antiviral and antibacterial properties. Recent studies indicate that ellagic acid may have anticarcinogenic effects by activating the p21 protein. Other reports indicate that ellagic acid also has potent antioxidant effects.
Essiac	This product is composed of four botanicals: burdock root, sheep sorrel root, slippery elm bark, and rhubarb root. The formula is consumed as a tea. Promoters claim that this product boosts the immune system, acts as a tonic, and treats cancer and HIV. However, no data or published clinical trials show efficacy for any claims made. Possible adverse effects include nausea, vomiting, diarrhea, constipation, hypoglycemia, and renal and hepatic toxicity with chronic consumption. There is a case report that indicates Essiac decreases clearance of camptothecan possibly because of the inhibition of cytochrome P-450 isoenzymes. Additional research is required to establish whether Essiac is safe and effective for any of its proposed claims.

Table 3-2
CONTINUED

Common Name	Mechanism of Action
Ginseng	Derived from the root of the plant. Patients take this supplement to improve athletic performance, strength and stamina, and as an immunostimulant for diabetes, cancer, HIV or acquired immunodeficiency syndrome (AIDS), and a variety of other conditions. The saponin glycosides, also known as ginsenosides, are thought to be responsible for *Panax ginseng*'s effects. Ginsenosides have both stimulatory and inhibitory effects on the central nervous system, alter cardio-vascular tone, increase humoral and cellular-dependent immunity, and may inhibit the growth of cancer in vitro. Use of *Panax ginseng* for chemoprevention reduces the incidence of chemically induced lung, liver, skin, and ovarian cancers in mice. Two case-controlled epidemiologic studies of Korean subjects suggest that *Panax ginseng* extract consumption reduces the incidence of all cancers. *Panax ginseng* is usually well tolerated, but insomnia, nausea, vomiting, and diarrhea have been reported. *Panax ginseng* may increase the hypoglycemic effect of insulin and sulfonylureas and possibly antagonize the effects of anticoagulants.
Graviola	Derived from a tree in the rain forests of Africa, South America, and Southeast Asia. The bark, leaves, root, and fruits have been used as traditional remedies in many countries. Extracts of graviola have been shown to have antiviral, antiparasitic, antirheumatic, astringent, emetic, antileishmanial, and cytotoxic effects. Graviola has also been shown to be effective against multidrug-resistant cancer cells line. There are no large scale studies in humans on the effects of graviola. Alkaloids extracted from graviola may cause neuronal dysfunction and degeneration leading to symptoms reminiscent of Parkinson's disease.

Table 3-2
CONTINUED

Common Name	Mechanism of Action
Green tea	Patients use this as a dietary beverage and to prevent and treat cancer, hyperlipidemia, hypertension, and atherosclerosis. The principal active constituent in green tea is epigallocatechin-3-gallate (EGCG), which accounts for 40% of the total polyphenol content of green tea extract. EGCG may inhibit enzymes involved in cell replication and DNA synthesis by interfering with cell-to-cell adhesion or via inhibition of intracellular communication pathways required for cell division. Studies of the chemopreventive activity of green tea indicated some positive results. Green tea polyphenols may reduce risk of prostate, breast, esophageal, lung, skin, pancreatic, and bladder cancers and oral leukoplakia. Administration of green tea before and during carcinogen treatment reduces the incidence and number of stomach and esophageal tumors in animals. Clinical research evaluating the effectiveness of green tea extracts to treat cancer is currently underway. Moderate intake of green tea appears to be safe.
Huang Lian	Derived from the root of the plant. This supplement is used in traditional Chinese medicine primarily for gastrointestinal complaints, diarrhea, hypertension, and bacterial and viral infections. Berberine and berberine-like alkaloids are thought responsible for its activity. Laboratory studies indicate that berberine induces morphological changes and internucleosomal DNA fragmentation in hepatoma cancer cells. Preliminary data has shown that Huang Lian suppresses cyclin B1 protein and causes cell cycle arrest at G2. It also interacts with acetylcholine and muscarinic receptors and inhibits cholinesterase. A phase I dose ranging study of Huang Lian in solid tumors is currently underway at Memorial Sloan-Kettering Cancer Center.

Table 3-2
CONTINUED

Common Name	Mechanism of Action
Indirubin	Indirubin is a compound isolated from Qing Dai, a dark blue powder prepared from the leaves of *Baphicacanthus cusia*. Preliminary studies indicate that indirubin is a potent inhibitor of cyclin-dependent kinases. It is effective in slowing proliferation of certain cancer cells, mainly through arresting the G2/M phase of the cell cycle.
Indole-3-carbinol	Indole-3-Carbinol (I3C) is a specific compound found in cruciferous vegetables including broccoli, cabbage, and cauliflower. Because diets high in these vegetables retard cancer growth in animals, I3C is thought to be a good candidate for cancer prevention. I3C is known to stimulate detoxification enzymes in the gut and liver. Several studies demonstrate that it can cause cell cycle arrest and apoptosis in cancer cells. In addition, it has ER-modulating effects and is thought to have potential value as a chemopreventive agent for breast cancer. I3C also down-regulates the expression of the estrogen-responsive genes *pS2* and cathepsin-D and up-regulates *BRAC1*. Other in vitro studies show that I3C inhibits the expression of cyclin-dependent kinase-6 and induces a G1 cell cycle arrest independent of ER signaling. One placebo-controlled trial shows that I3C is effective in treating precancerous cervical dysplasia. I3C is generally well tolerated when taken orally. Certain studies suggest I3C may promote tumor growth in animals that have been exposed to carcinogens, but the potential risk has never been documented in humans. Because it may induce cytochrome P-450, I3C has potential interactions with other medications.
Lentinan	A polysaccharide derived from the mycelium of shiitake mushroom. It is considered a biological response modifier. Lentinan's active polysaccharide 1,3-glucan is not cytotoxic but seems to enhance

Table 3-2
CONTINUED

Common Name	Mechanism of Action
Lentinan *continued*	T-helper cell function, increase stimulation of interleukin, interferon, and normal killer cells. In addition to antitumor activity, it also possesses immune-regulatory effects, antiviral activity, antimicrobial properties. and cholesterol-lowering effects.
Maitake	Derived from the cap and stem of maitake mushroom. The active constituent is thought to be a glucan polysaccharide. Maitake is thought to exert its effects through its ability to activate various effector cells such as macrophages, natural killer cells, T cells, IL-1, and superoxide anions. In a small noncontrolled study in cancer patients, tumor regression or significant symptom improvements were observed in half of the subjects who took maitake extract. Some studies reveal a hypoglycemic effect following administration of maitake extract. Research is underway to test maitake's anticancer effects in humans.
Mistletoe	Derived from the aerial parts of the plant. Patients use mistletoe preparations for a variety of conditions including cancer, HIV, hepatitis, and degenerative joint disease. Polypeptides including lectins and viscotoxins are thought responsible for in vitro immune stimulant and tumor inhibition activity. Lectins induce macrophage cytotoxicity, stimulate phagocytosis of immune cells, increase cytokine secretion (TNF-α, IL-1, IL-2, IL-6), and enhance cytotoxicity effects on various cell lines in vitro. A recent epidemiologic study suggests a possible survival advantage following treatment with mistletoe. Controlled clinical trials in humans yielded mixed results. There is an ongoing trial on using mistletoe extract and gemcitabine for the treatment of solid tumors.

Table 3-2
CONTINUED

Common Name	Mechanism of Action
Noni	Derived from the fruit, leaves, and roots of the tree. Noni is a traditional Polynesian remedy for a variety of conditions including cancer, hypertension, and diabetes. Several polysaccharides, anthraquinones, and alkaloids are thought responsible for its activity. The fruit juice contains noni-ppt, a polysaccharide-rich substance, which enhances survival of inbred Lewis Lung carcinoma bearing mice. Noni-ppt is thought to act by an immunomodulatory mechanism. It increases nitric oxide production from murine peritoneal macrophages and stimulates the release of cytokines, IL-1, and TNF-α from human peripheral mononuclear cells. No human clinical trials evaluating noni for any proposed claims are published. Due to the high sugar content in the fruit juice, diabetics should use noni juice with caution.
Pau d'Arco	Derived from the bark of the tree. This herb has been used traditionally to treat cancer and infections. No clinical studies support its use for these claims. The quinone compounds of the herb are known to possess toxic effects. Use of this product may increase the activity of anticoagulants.
PC SPES	PC SPES is a natural product comprised of eight herbs: reishi, baikal skullcap, dyer's woad, chrysanthemum, saw palmetto, *Panax ginseng*, licorice, and rabdosia. Patients use this supplement to treat prostate cancer. In vitro testing reveals suppression of human tumor cell lines, including androgen-sensitive and -insensitive prostate cancer. Use of PC SPES brings about significant decrease in androgen and PSA levels in human clinical trials. It is thought that PC SPES contains phytoestrogens and other undefined components that contribute to its activity. Recent concerns about product contamination with warfarin and alprazolam resulted in a voluntary recall of PC SPES by the manufacturer.

Table 3-2
CONTINUED

Common Name	Mechanism of Action
Soy	Soybeans contain various proteins, vitamins, and minerals, as well as significant amounts of isoflavones (e.g., genistein, daidzein, and glycitein), and are a good source of fiber. Isoflavones are considered phytoestrogens and exhibit both selective estrogen receptor modulator activity and non-hormonal effects. Clinical data suggest that soy isoflavones are no more effective than placebo for treating menopausal symptoms in patients with breast cancer. Epidemiologic, animal, and in vitro data suggest that soy may be used as an alternative to conventional hormone replacement therapy to treat menopausal symptoms, but with questionable efficacy. Other data suggest that soy may slow bone density loss and prevent breast cancer, but clinical results are inconsistent. Evidence suggesting that soy proteins have a protective effect against prostate cancer is primarily epidemiologic or in vitro. It is unknown whether isoflavones influence hormone-dependent cancers. However, one epidemiological report suggests dietary soy can increase risk of bladder cancer. Numerous studies indicate that soy lowers total cholesterol levels. Animal and human studies reveal that soy protein can decrease LDL cholesterol, inhibit LDL oxidation, and possibly increase HDL cholesterol.
Sun soup	This is a proprietary product that contains, soybean, shiitake mushroom, mung bean, red date, scallion, garlic, lentil bean, leek, hawthorn fruit, onion, American ginseng, angelica root, licorice, dandelion root, senegal root, ginger, olive, sesame seed, and parsley. Patients use this supplement in conjunction with conventional therapies to prevent and treat cancer and HIV/AIDS and communicate weight gain, and as an immunostimulant. This product exhibits antitumor activity in animals. Data in phase I/II studies suggest improvements in survival, Karnofsky Performance Scale Score, and objective tumor regression when administered concurrently with conventional therapies for stage III and IV non-small cell lung cancer. Larger randomized studies are underway to substantiate this data.

Table 3-2
CONTINUED

Common Name	Mechanism of Action
Turmeric	Derived from the rhizome and root. This supplement is routinely used as a spice and coloring agent. Curcuminoids (curcumin) and volatile oil found in turmeric are partly responsible for the therapeutic activities. Curcuminoids induce glutathione S-transferase and are potent inhibitors of cytochrome P-450. Turmeric acts as a free radical scavenger and antioxidant, inhibiting lipid peroxidation and oxidative DNA damage. Although in vitro and animal studies suggest antiproliferative and preventative effects against cancer, human data are lacking. Recent animal studies indicate that dietary turmeric may inhibit the antitumor action of chemotherapeutic agents such as cyclophosphamide in treating breast cancer. More research is necessary, but it may be advisable for breast cancer patients undergoing chemotherapy to limit intake of turmeric and turmeric-containing foods

AIDS = acquired immunodeficiency syndrome; DNA = deoxyribonucleic acid; ER = estrogen receptor; HIV = human immunodeficiency virus; IL = interleukin; TCM = traditional Chinese medicine; TNF = tumor necrosis factor

READINGS AND RESOURCES

1. Memorial Sloan-Kettering Cancer Center. About herbs, botanical & other products. http://www.mskcc.org/aboutherbs (accessed March 8, 2005).

4

Botanicals, Cancer, and Herb–Drug Interactions

ANALYSIS, STANDARDIZATION, AND REGULATION

Herbalists identify herbs by the organoleptic method, which involves the use of all human senses. To identify an herb, the trained herbalist examines its external appearance, smells its aroma, touches it to determine surface texture, chews it looking for the special balance of taste, and may even listen to the snap of a twig to estimate its moisture content. These skills are passed down through generations and are still in use today when more reliable equipment is not available.

Advances in botanical science enable more definitive identification methods involving examining the histomorphology of the microscopic cellular structure of plants. In addition, techniques such as thin-layer chromatography (TLC), high-performance liquid chromatography (HPLC), gas chromatography (GC), mass spectrometry (MS), capillary electrophoresis (CE), and ultraviolet–visible (UV-VIS) spectrophotometry are commonly employed to recognize the chemical fingerprints of botanicals (Table 4-1).

Advances in plant genetics have ushered the authentication of botanicals into a new era. Microarray chips and other related technologies have been developed to identify a species based on the plant's genetic makeup. This has significant impact on the quality control of botanicals in the future, as inexpensive portable test kits will be available for quick authentication of samples.

Standardization remains a problem in contemporary botanical products. Unlike synthetic chemicals produced in a lab with US Food and Drug Administration (FDA) oversight, botanical products may contain active components that vary from batch to batch depending on conditions of cultivation and processing. There are reports on super- or subpotent products in the market. Survey of ginseng sup-

Table 4-1

MARKER COMPOUNDS FOR SOME COMMON BOTANICALS

Botanical	Marker Compound	Test
Black cohosh	Triterpene glucosides	HPLC
Cat's claw	Oxindole alkaloids	CE
Cayenne	Capsaicin	HPLC
Clover	Isoflavones	HPLC
Echinacea	Echinacoside	HPLC
Feverfew	Parthenolide	CE
Garlic	Adenosine	CE
Ginkgo biloba	Flavonglycosides	HPLC
Ginseng	Ginsenosides	HPLC
Goldenseal	Berberine	CE
Grape skin extract	Resveratrol	HPLC
Green tea	Catechins	HPLC
Hawthorn	Vitexin	HPLC
Kava kava	Kava lactones	HPLC
Licorice	Glycyrrhizic acid	CE
Wild yam	Diosgenin	HPLC
Milk thistle	Silymarin	UV-VIS
Peppermint	Menthol	GC
Rose hip	Ascorbic acid	HPLC
Saw palmetto	Phytosterols	GC
Senna	Sennosides	HPLC
Soy	Isoflavones	HPLC
St.John's wort	Hypericin	HPLC

CE = capillary electrophoresis; GC = gas chromatography; HPLC = high-performance liquid chromatography; UV-VIS = ultraviolet–visible spectrophotometry.

plements from different companies indicates that the actual amount of the active components ranges from 10 to over 200% of the labeled quantity.

Methods to standardize commercial preparations are required to ensure consistent quality and ingredients among batches. For the identification and quality control components of standardization, the presence and concentration of the most abundant active constituents is evaluated. Where active components are unknown, a surrogate chemical marker is used. A standardized botanical product must contain a predetermined amount of this marker in every batch. *Ginkgo biloba* tablets, for example, are standardized to contain 24% ginkgo flavone glycosides and 6% terpene lactones. Not all manufacturers conform to these standards.

The regulation of herbal preparations varies by country, ranging from no specific laws to highly regulated legislation. Several European countries regard and treat herbal products as prescription drugs. In Japan, Kampo products, which consist of classic TCM herbal formulas, are restricted to use by physicians trained in Western medicine. Kampo products are covered by Japan's national health insurance system.

Since 1994, botanicals in the United States have been regulated as dietary supplements under the Dietary Supplement Health and Education Act (DSHEA). Unlike prescription drugs or other over-the-counter remedies, the FDA may not review botanical products for safety and effectiveness (see Chapter 1). Manufacturers must indicate that their product is not intended to diagnose, treat, cure, or prevent any disease. However, they may claim benefits related to a nutrient-deficiency problem or describe how the product can affect people's structure, function, or general well-being.

Although the FDA does not evaluate botanical products, it has the legislative power to ban botanical products if proven unsafe for human consumption. A recent example is ephedra, a product used as a stimulant and for weight loss, which was banned in April 2004 because of side effects arising from misuse and abuse. As growing numbers of adverse effects from botanicals have surfaced, a strong lobbying effort has been made to tighten regulation of the sale and use of botanicals.

CONTAMINANTS

Pesticides, heavy metals, microbials, and extraneous matter are the most common contaminants found in botanical preparations. Although most commercial herb farms use only approved pesticides, residual pesticides may be harmful in high concentrations, especially in crops grown in contaminated soil. There is evidence that toxic levels of the long-banned pesticide dichlorodiphenyltrichloroethane

(DDT) can still be found in some imported botanical products. Manufacturers of these products must include routine screening for organophosphorus and organochlorine pesticides as part of the quality control process.

Heavy metals such as lead, mercury, and arsenic are found in botanicals grown in soil with high concentrations of these metals naturally or as a result of industrial runoff. Excessive amounts of heavy metals or related compounds may be added intentionally to traditional botanical formulas to enhance therapeutic effect. Such products are unsafe for consumption, especially by young children and pregnant women.

All botanical products are exposed to microbials during cultivation, handling, or storage. The presence of microbials does not necessarily imply inferiority in the raw material. However, pathogenic organisms in the final product as a result of improper cleaning, sterilization, or packaging are not uncommon and could be detrimental. The US Pharmacopeia requires testing of supplements for viable cultures of *Staphylococcus aureus, Escherichia coli, Pseudomonas aeruginosa, Candida albicans, Aspergillus niger,* and *Salmonella* species.

Extraneous matter is another possible contaminant. Compounds such as aflatoxin and mycotoxin from molds, insect parts, animal

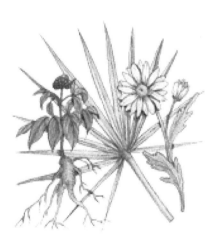

Figure 4-1 PC-SPES, shown to decrease PSA levels, was recalled following discovery of product contamination.

excreta, broken glass, and dirt have been found in botanical products produced under poor manufacturing conditions. Chemical solvents and unlabeled pharmaceuticals have been discovered in many imported herbal formulas, a problem traced back to poor quality control, solvent recycling, and the common practice in some countries of mixing Western pharmaceutical drugs with traditional herbal formulas. Unfortunately, such combinations can cause drug interactions or allergic reactions. A well-known example is the botanical compound PC SPES, used in prostate cancer research. PC SPES was found to be contaminated with a female hormone, a tranquilizer, and anti-inflammatory drugs and was forced off the market even though the formula showed efficacy in clinical trials.

Toxicities

Despite spotty standardization and contamination issues, botanical products are generally regarded as safer than pharmaceuticals. Indeed, in Hong Kong, where the majority of people use herbs, only 0.2% of general medical admissions to a major hospital were due to adverse effects of herbal medicine, compared with 4.4% caused by Western pharmaceuticals. However, this does not mean botanicals are absolutely safe, as the general public tends to believe. Some of the most toxic substances known are derived from plants. Botanicals can be toxic to specific organs or cause allergic or idiosyncratic responses. Listed below are examples of such toxicities.

Nephrotoxicity

Plants that contain aristolochic acid can damage the kidneys if ingested in excessive amounts. Several cases of nephrotoxicity were reported in women in Belgium following ingestion of high doses of herbal diuretic preparations used for weight loss. The major ingredient of these preparations turned out to be *Aristolochia fangchi* root, which contains aristolochic acid. This substance is also known to be carcinogenic. Other cases of toxicity using substitution species, including *Aristolochia manshuriensis* and *Stephania tetrandra*, have been reported in France, the United Kingdom, China, and Japan. Substitution of species with similar activities is a common practice in traditional medicine and can also be caused by misidentification. The use of botanicals that contain aristolochic acid is discouraged.

Hepatotoxicity

Apiole is an irritant found in the volatile oil of parsley, prolonged use of which can cause liver damage. Pyrrolizidine alkaloids are hepatotoxic and are found in species such as *Crotalaria*, *Heliotropium*, and *Senecio*. Common herbs such as borage, comfrey, coltsfoot, and echinacea also have small amounts of a less toxic form of pyrrolizidine. Lignans from chaparral also have been linked to liver toxicity. Patients with preexisting liver conditions should avoid prolonged use and high doses of these botanicals.

Cardiotoxicity

Many botanicals contain cardiac glycosides. When used appropriately, such botanicals have provided valuable drugs to treat cardiovascular diseases. For example, digoxin, the drug of choice for heart failure, is extracted from the herb foxglove. Other common cardiac glycoside–containing botanicals include aconite, ginseng, hawthorn, and licorice. Overconsumption of these botanicals or concurrent use with prescription drugs can cause adverse effects similar to toxicity from digitalis, including bradycardia and cardiac arrest. In addition, there are problems related to contamination and adulteration. Traces of digitalis have been found in products labeled as "plantain" and "Siberian ginseng." Botanical supplements harvested in poorly controlled environments are especially prone to such errors.

Neurotoxicity

Some botanicals exhibit neural activities. For example, the herbs guarana and ephedra affect the central nervous system (CNS). Excessive amounts of these herbs can cause palpitation, agitation, and, in extreme cases, seizure and death. Botanicals like St. John's wort and kava kava, used as antidepressants and tranquilizers, may produce sedative effects and should not be used with prescription drugs that have similar activity.

Phototoxicity

Photosensitivity has been associated with the consumption of plants containing compounds such as furocoumarins or psoralens from the families Umbelliferae (including parsley and celery) and Rutaceae (including bergamot and citrus fruits). Phototoxicity reactions have been reported after topical application of bergamot oil and ingestion of a large quantity of celery soup. Some have suffered severe skin burns when exposed to the sun after using *Psoralea corylifolia* ("Bu-gu-zhi"), a popular Chinese herb that contains psoralen. Patients treated with radiation therapy are particularly vulnerable to this effect.

Carcinogenicity

Some plant compounds are known to be carcinogenic. For example, beta-asarone found in calamus oil, estragole in the oils of tarragon, fennel and basil, and safrole in sassafras oil can cause cancer in animals. The culinary use of these products as spices appears to be harmless, due to the small amount of intake. However, health care professionals and patients should be aware of these effects when using these botanicals in greater doses as supplements.

Herb-Drug Interactions

Botanicals can affect the function of other drugs when used concomitantly. The two major interactions are pharmacokinetic interactions that occur when an herb affects the absorption, distribution, metabolism, and excretion of other drugs or herbs and vice versa and pharmacodynamic interactions that occur when an herb affects the pharmacological properties of other drugs or herbs and vice versa.

The interaction between grapefruit juice and other drugs was discovered accidentally when grapefruit juice was used as a control in pharmacokinetic studies. The studies found that grapefruit juice, but not orange juice, can cause a threefold increase in the bioavailability of certain drugs. Subsequently, it was found that compounds called furacoumarins, which are abundant in grapefruit juice, can bind irreversibly with an enzyme called cytochrome P-450 (CYP) 3A4 in the intestinal wall. Normally, CYP 3A4 slows down or inhibits the absorption of many drugs at this point. The inhibition of CYP 3A4, conversely, allows the absorption of such drugs in larger amount. The increase in bioavailability can increase the toxicity of drugs, such as tacrolimus and cyclosporin, that have narrow margins of safety.

CYP 3A4 is also present in the liver where many drugs are metabolized. Herbs like St. John's wort can induce this microsomal enzyme and cause a decrease in the serum level of other drugs that are metabolized by the same enzyme. One report indicated that serum level of irinotecan can be reduced by 40% when a patient takes St. John's wort concurrently.

P-Glycoprotein

P-glycoprotein is a cell-surface protein that transports drugs and other substances across the cell membrane. It is found in the colon, small intestine, adrenal glands, kidney, and liver. It is also expressed by tumor cells and is responsible for drug resistance during chemotherapy by increasing the elimination of cytotoxic agents. Botanicals such as St. John's wort can elevate the expression of intestinal P-glycoprotein, thereby decreasing the bioavailability and effects of certain chemotherapeutic agents.

Anticoagulants or Antiplatelets

Numerous botanicals contain coumarin or coumarin-like substances. They are relatively benign until coumarin is converted to dicumarol by microbial actions. Dicumarol can inhibit the action of vitamin K in the liver and potentially can cause prolonged coagulation. Warfarin, a commonly used anticoagulant, is the synthetic analog of dicumarol. Warfarin dosing requires careful titration. A dose that is too low can result in thrombosis and too high can cause hemorrhage. Botanicals that contain coumarin may have synergistic effects with concurrent use of warfarin, causing excessive bleeding. Other botanicals, including ginger, ginseng, garlic, feverfew, and ginkgo, that have antiplatelet effects may cause postoperative hemorrhage. For example, large

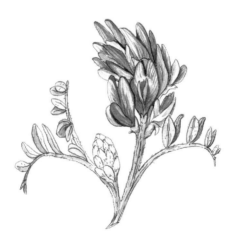

Figure 4-2 Astragalus is used for its immunostimulating properties.

amounts of garlic are associated with increased bleeding during surgical procedures such as transurethral resection of the prostate and augmentation mammoplasty.

Phytoestrogens

Botanicals such as red clover, soy, Dong Guai, and wild yam are known to have weak estrogenic effects. Patients with estrogen-receptor-positive breast cancer or other hormone-sensitive cancers should avoid using these botanicals as they may stimulate the proliferation of cancer cells (see Chapter 11).

Immune-Enhancing Botanicals

Botanicals known to have immunostimulant effects may cause complications in transplant patients and in patients on immunosuppressants. Studies suggest that Astragalus can reverse cyclophosphamide-induced immune suppression. Echinacea may have similar properties.

5

Diet and Nutrition

Diet is one of the very few ways that cancer patients can play a role in their recovery. Following diagnosis and a treatment plan, the first question typically asked by patients concerns what they should and should not eat to help keep their disease at bay. Those in remission want to know how to change their diet to help preclude recurrence. Family members seize nutrition as a major opportunity to help their loved one. Patients and family members appropriately see food as an opportunity to help maintain strength throughout treatment, reduce the toxicity of chemotherapy or radiation, enhance quality of life, and facilitate comfort during end-stage disease.

Although hospital dieticians and nutritionists can provide expert, detailed help, patients typically seek guidance from their physicians. Often that advice is "eat what you want." Even where clinically appropriate, this advice does not facilitate the patient's and family's desire to play a role in working toward remission. Often they turn to books and the Internet, where they find an abundance of information. However, many find books such as the American Cancer Society's *Eating Well, Staying Well During and After Cancer*, or the National Cancer Institute's Web site section "Nutrition in Cancer Care" less attractive than headlines about dietary "cures."

This chapter provides basic information about nutritional guidelines in cancer care, reviews organic foods and other issues often raised by patients, and briefly describes a few popular bogus dietary "cures."

GENERAL DIETARY RECOMMENDATIONS

The World Cancer Research Fund and the American Institute for Cancer Research (AICR) published the landmark report "Food, Nutrition and the Prevention of Cancer: A Global Perspective" in 1997, the culmination of the work of over 100 international experts who evaluated all available data on the link between diet and cancer.

Their conclusions and recommendations, further substantiated by major research since that time, recommend plant-based diets. These include a variety of vegetables, fruits, whole grains and legumes, lean sources of protein from poultry and fish, and low- and nonfat dairy products. These foods contain phytochemicals and antioxidants that neutralize carcinogens before they damage healthy cells and that may help normalize cells early in the carcinogenic process. They also are naturally high in fiber, which is similarly protective against cancer.

The American Dietetic Association and other nutrition-concerned organizations have worked to revamp the flawed US Department of Agriculture (USDA) Food Guide Pyramid, which has failed to acknowledge the important difference between refined and whole grain foods. Whole grains will become part of the new Food Guide Pyramid under development by the USDA as of this writing. The Food Guide Pyramid from Walter C. Willett, MD at the Harvard School of Public Health provides excellent guidelines.

The evidence is convincing that diets high in fruits, vegetables, and unrefined grains reduce the risk of a variety of cancers as well as heart disease, stroke, hypertension, and diabetes. The AICR pamphlet "Moving Toward a Plant-Based Diet: Menus and Recipes for Cancer Prevention" is useful for patients and available from the AICR.

Many patients retain their ability to eat normally during treatment; others change their intake around the days of therapy because of related side effects. For those eager to do what they can to help themselves, cancer patients should be encouraged to follow this approach. For modifications and assistance with gastrointestinal problems (see Chapter 17), symptom management, food preparation to facilitate swallowing and digestion, and so on, a clinical oncology dietitian should become involved. The references noted above and at the end of this chapter also may be recommended to patients.

PESTICIDES AND ORGANIC FOODS

Toxins associated with pesticides used in farming are of major concern to many patients. Typically, patients hear or read that they should consume only organic produce to avoid the cancer-causing pesticides in standard commercial produce. However, claims made by marketers of organic produce, which is more expensive than produce farmed without pesticides, are overblown. According to the American Cancer Society, environmental factors, including chemicals and radiation as well as smoking, diet, and infectious diseases, probably cause three-quarters of all cancer cases in the United States. Among these, tobacco use, unhealthy diet, and insufficient physical activity affect cancer risk more than do the trace levels of pollutants found in food, drinking water, and air.

Public concern tends to focus on pesticides, even though known carcinogen exposure is at such low levels that risks are negligible. High doses have been shown to cause cancer in animals, but the very low concentrations in foods are not associated with increased cancer risk. The important message for patients is that people who eat more fruits and vegetables, possibly contaminated with trace amounts of pesticides, generally have lower cancer risks than those who eat few fruits and vegetables.

But, patients ask, are "organic" foods— those grown without pesticides or genetic modification—better? No research demonstrates that they are. Moreover, foods produced organically appear to be virtually indistinguishable from foods produced in the standard agricultural fashion. According to the USDA, "No distinctions should be made between organically and non-organically produced products in terms of quality, appearance, or safety."

Research does not support the claims of organic food marketers and proponents that their foods are safer due to lower levels of pesticide residue. Pesticide levels in the US food supply, standard or organic, are found only in trace amounts. Moreover, a study by the Institute of Food Technologists' Expert Panel on Food Safety and Nutrition found that pesticides may reduce health risks by destroying microorganisms and preventing the growth of harmful molds and other organisms that produce toxic substances.

Nor are organic foods more nutritious, as the nutrient content of plants is based primarily on heredity. Of particular importance, most studies conducted over the past four decades found similar pesticide levels in foods designated organic and those that were not. For example, *Consumer Reports* in 1988 published their study of a thousand pounds of tomatoes, peaches, green bell peppers, and apples. The produce had been purchased in five US cities and then was tested for synthetic pesticides. Traces were detected in 77% of conventional foods and 25% of organically labeled foods, but the level of pesticides was similar in both. Only one sample of each exceeded the federal limit. Pesticides are reduced or eliminated by washing them with detergent. Organic foods require similar preparation to destroy some of the microorganisms that were not eliminated by pesticides.

XENOESTROGENS

A related common concern is that agricultural chemicals are xenoestrogens, which can remain in human adipose tissue, such as the breast, for years. A large well-designed study examined the possible relationship between prolonged xenoestrogen exposure and breast cancer initiation. Results were published in the *New England Journal of Medicine* in 1997; researchers found no link between blood levels of pesticide metabolites and breast cancer risk. Many other studies also addressed the breast cancer–chemical toxin hypothesis; the American Cancer Society describes as "weak and inconsistent" the evidence that pollutants and pesticide residues increase cancer risk.

GROWTH HORMONE AND ANTIBIOTICS

Patients often ask if they should avoid dairy products, commercial meats, and poultry because of artificial growth hormones and antibiotics administered to the animals. Specifically, they worry that growth hormones will increase the risk of hormone-sensitive cancers. Commercial dairy products, in particular, anecdotally are suspected of increasing the risk of breast cancer because of circulating levels of insulin-like growth factors (IGFs) and the presence of recombinant bovine growth hormone (rBGH). To date, no clinical evidence supports this hypothesis.

DIGESTIVE ENZYMES

Pancreatin and other digestive enzymes are routinely prescribed for patients with pancreatic or other digestive insufficiencies. Digestive enzyme preparations also are available in health food stores as dietary supplements, where patients read that these enzymes help fight cancer via their ability to uncouple cancer-causing antigen–antibody complexes and by enhancing immune function. Some clinical evidence supports these claims, but the data are far from definitive.

Digestive enzymes can be useful because they may enable more complete extraction of vital nutrients from food. However, they can produce side effects and interact with pharmaceuticals (see Chapter 4), and those sold as food supplements may be contaminated.

JUICING

Juice extractors dice food and then spin to separate the juice from fiber-containing pulp. Juicing is touted as a more efficient means of consuming the nutrients in fruits, vegetables, and enzymes. This may be true for the phytochemicals in the liquid portion of the juice, but sustained absence of fiber is not desirable. Fiber is more than the soluble and insoluble fractions of plant foods that aid in bowel function; fibers also serve as the substrate for the beneficial gut bacteria that line the human gastrointestinal tract. The digestion and metabolism of fiber by these bacteria yield byproducts with cell-protective and anticancer properties. Inadequate fibrous content deprives the consumer of an array of beneficial compounds, and ongoing food science research inevitably will identify other disease-fighting phytochemicals in the bacterial degradation of plant components.

Juicing is fine as a complement to, but not a substitute for, standard fruit and vegetable intake. It may also increase calorie intake and assist hydration for those in need. If used to extreme, however, juicing may increase antioxidant intake well beyond the recommended dietary allowance (RDA). This raises the unresolved concern that high antioxidant intake may interfere with chemotherapy and radi-

Table 5-1
RAW FOODS OR COOKED?

Popular Internet sites promote raw foods, sometimes in association with juicing recommendations and the sale of juicers. Many cancer patients come to believe that cooking destroys the value of foods and that raw food intake will best help control their disease. Raw food diets, in fact, are not scientifically justified and can be counterproductive, as cooking is needed to destroy bacteria, denature proteins ,and facilitate digestion. Cancer patients often require the softer, easier to chew, and more digestible foods that cooking produces.

ation, which is based on the underlying question of whether these therapies work through an antioxidant or free radical mechanism (see Chapter 6).

POPULAR DIETARY "CANCER TREATMENTS"

Patients often translate from prevention to cure, assuming that, because certain foods help prevent cancer, they also can treat established disease. Patients need be reminded that no diet itself can cure cancer, despite commercial claims to the contrary. The promotion of a particular diet as a viable treatment option is appealing to patients who do not recognize its dangers. Patients need to hear that delaying treatment to give the "special diet" a chance to work enables additional tumor growth and, eventually, more advanced, less treatable disease.

Some questionable dietary treatments require that patients consume only a single item. Examples include the grape cure and wheatgrass cancer therapy. The former consists of restricting one's diet to grapes, the latter to liquefied grass. Both still have proponents, and wheatgrass therapy clinics now exist in Florida and Puerto Rico. A no-dairy diet is in vogue as of this writing, attracting notice especially among patients with breast cancer, who fear that hormones fed to cows result in dairy products that encourage the growth of cancer cells.

Macrobiotics

Developed by Japanese philosopher George Ohsawa in the 1930s, macrobiotics remains a popular system of healing through diet and natural medicine. It incorporates the yin–yang principles of balance central to traditional Chinese medicine (see Chapter 2) and emphasizes spiritual and social aspects of living as well as specific foods and cooking techniques. This system has its own unique concepts of the pathophysiology of disease and uses unconventional diagnostic techniques such as iridology. Because these are unsound, disease may go undiagnosed or misdiagnosed. Macrobiotic diagnostic procedures also may lead to false diagnoses, which set the stage for later displays of apparently cured cancer patients.

The original, severely restrictive macrobiotic diet caused serious nutritional deficiencies, after which the diet was amended. The current version has positive aspects, including emphasis on whole grains for 50 to 60% and vegetables for 25 to 30% of daily intake. Remaining calories are obtained from soy and other legumes, sea vegetables, miso soup, and small amounts of white meat fish and shellfish. Fruit is limited to a few times per week.

Prohibited are dairy products, meats, eggs, tomatoes, white potatoes, coffee, sugar, and all processed foods. These are not unreasonable recommendations for good health, but strict adherence leaves cancer patients lacking micronutrients such as iron, zinc, B_{12}, and calcium. Caloric intake also may be inadequate, and this diet does not lend itself to overcoming treatment-related side effects. Patients require sufficient protein to help rebuild damaged tissues, and macrobiotics may leave patients protein deficient. The diet recommends against using vitamin or mineral supplements.

This is also a difficult and time-consuming diet to follow, requiring calculation of one's geographic location, the time of year, and so on to determine permitted foods. Scientific evidence does not support the macrobiotic diet as a cancer cure, nor is there support for the idea of balancing yin–yang aspects of food with the yin or yang of the patient's particular cancer. Further, macrobiotic principles produce recommendations that are contrary to established nutrition science. For example, tomatoes and tomato products, which are important components of a healthy Mediterranean diet and also protect against prostate cancer, are not permitted on the macrobiotic plan because they are too yin. Principles conceptualized by ancient thinkers to structure their understanding of health and disease are not always consistent with more recent understanding.

Vegetarianism

There are three types of vegetarian diets. Ovolactovegetarians include dairy and eggs in their plant-based diet. Lactovegetarians include dairy products. Vegans eliminate all animal foods, including fish, and concentrate exclusively on grains, vegetables, fruits, beans, nuts, seeds, and vegetable oils. Of the three approaches, the vegan diet carries the greatest risk of micronutrient deficiency. All vegetarians risk vitamin B_{12} deficiency from the avoidance of animal proteins, but vegans also risk calcium and vitamin D deficiency from the absence of dairy products. The obvious remedy for these concerns is supplementation with either of these individual nutrients or the use of a 100% RDA multivitamin.

Vegetarianism presents a risk for cancer patients only if they fail to consume a balanced diet with adequate protein intake, supplementing with the necessary micronutrients. As with macrobiotics, vegetarianism is not a cure for cancer. Research has documented the ability of low-fat vegetarian diets to lower the risk for a variety of diseases including hypercholesterolemia, heart disease, diabetes, hypertension obesity, and some forms of cancer. Conversely, a vegetarian diet that includes whole fat milk, butter, French fries, and potato chips probably will increase the risk of these diseases. A vegetarian diet in any of its manifestations can be health promoting if approached with due diligence to including a variety of foods with appropriate supplementation.

METABOLIC DIETARY REGIMENS

Hoxsey Therapy

Comprised of herbal tonics and restrictive diet, this regimen is promoted as a viable alternative to mainstream cancer treatment. The Hoxsey treatment is illegal in the United States but available at clinics in Tijuana, Mexico. According to inventor Harry Hoxsey (1901–1974), a self-taught healer, the key "brown" tonic contains potassium iodide and multiple herbs (licorice, red clover, burdock root, stillingia root, barberry, cascara, pokeroot, prickly ash bark, and buckthorn bark).

The diet eliminates pork, vinegar, tomatoes, pickles, carbonated drinks, alcohol, bleached flour, sugar, and salt, and emphasizes iron, calcium, vitamin C, yeast supplements, and grape juice. Other supplements also may be included in the regimen. Hoxsey claimed that his treatment detoxifies the body, strengthens the immune system, balances body chemistry, and helps the body digest and excrete tumors.

Gerson Regimen

Developed by Max Gerson in the 1930s, this regimen involves a strict diet, coffee enemas, and various supplements including Laetrile,

- Hoxsey was convicted numerous times for practicing medicine without a license.
- The National Cancer Institute evaluated 77 case reports submitted by Hoxsey and concluded that none showed efficacy.
- The US government reported that the 400 patients Hoxsey claimed to have cured never had cancer, were cured before receiving his treatment, still had cancer, or had died from the disease.
- No clinical data support the value of this therapy, and patients should be urged not to use this method.

which is illegal in the United States. The regimen is available at clinics in Mexico and elsewhere. The current Gerson Institute Web site identifies 49 cancers and degenerative diseases cured with their regimen. The diet emphasizes fresh fruit and vegetable juice, high carbohydrate and potassium, no sodium or fat, and low animal protein and is sometimes supplemented with exogenous digestive enzymes. Again reflecting early concepts in traditional Chinese and Indian medicine (see Chapter 2), this regimen claims to address the cause of cancer by detoxifying the system and stimulating metabolism so that the body can heal itself.

However, coffee enemas have caused infections, dangerous electrolyte deficiencies, and death. Despite proponent claims of recovery rates as high as 70 to 90%, case reviews by the National Cancer Institute and the New York County Medical Society found no evidence of benefit against cancer.

Livingston-Wheeler Therapy

Virginia Livingston-Wheeler based her treatment on the discarded early twentieth-century theory that cancer is caused by the bacterium *Progenitor cryptocides*. Believing that weakened immune systems allow the bacterium to grow, she developed a regimen to counteract the deficiency and stimulate immune response. That treatment program is still available at the San Diego, California clinic that bears her name. It includes a strict vegetarian diet, BCG vaccine, coffee enemas, autogenous vaccine, vitamins, antibiotics, antioxidants, and nutritional and supportive counseling.

Dr Livingston-Wheeler died in 1990, the same year that the California Department of Health ordered the clinic to stop administering the vaccine, which had been made from the patient's own urine or blood. Metabolic diets may result in nutrient deficiencies, and repeated use of coffee enemas is linked to deaths from infection and electrolyte imbalance. A self-selected, matched cohort, prospective study of patients at the Livingston-Wheeler Clinic and a mainstream comprehensive cancer center found no difference in survival between groups and consistently lower quality of life in the Livingston-Wheeler cohort. Despite the absence of benefit and documented toxicities, patients still seek this therapy for cancer, arthritis, allergies, and acquired immunodeficiency syndrome (AIDS).

READINGS AND RESOURCES

1. Harvard School of Public Health. http://www.hsph.harvard.edu/nutrition-source/pyramids.html (accessed March 10, 2005).
2. Hunter DJ, Hankinson SE, Laden F, et al. Plasma organochlorine levels and the risk of breast cancer. N Engl J Med 1997;337:1253–8.
3. National Cancer Institute. http://www.cancer.gov/cancertopics/pdq/supportivecare/nutrition/healthprofessional (accessed March 10, 2005).

6

Vitamins and Dietary Supplements

Vitamins and supplements are by far the most popular form of complementary and alternative medicine used in the United States. The Slone Epidemiology Center at Boston University conducts ongoing telephone surveys that provide current population-based information on the use of all medications in the United States, including vitamins and minerals, herbal preparations, and other supplements, as well as prescription and over-the-counter drugs. The 2002 Slone Survey report showed that vitamins and minerals are used by 40% of the population. Multiple vitamins, vitamin E, vitamin C, and calcium are most commonly used. Only 6% use vitamin supplements under physician recommendation.

In theory, a balanced diet should produce adequate nutritional intake. However, cancer patients are more vulnerable to nutritional deficiency because of decreased appetite, poor absorption, or side effects of cancer treatment. They may require supplementation. A multivitamin or mineral product approved by the US Department of Agriculture (USDA) should be recommended. Proprietary vitamin products from some vendors lack essential constituents or contain unnecessary and undesirable ingredients. This chapter includes discussion of supplement regulation and quality control. The issue of antioxidants is also discussed, and a summary of vitamins and other supplements of particular promise or under study is provided.

REGULATION AND QUALITY CONTROL

In the United States, vitamins are regulated as dietary supplements under the Dietary Supplement Health Education Act (DSHEA) of 1994.

Because vitamins and other supplements are not regulated by the US Food and Drug Administration (FDA), the quality of available products differs substantially across manufacturers. Some vitamins contain too much or too little of the labeled ingredient. Others are manufactured under such poorly controlled conditions that active components cannot properly be absorbed. Vitamins and other sup-

> The Dietary Supplement Health and Education Act defines a dietary supplement as "a product (other than tobacco) that is intended to supplement the diet which bears or contains one or more of the following dietary ingredients: a vitamin, a mineral, an herb or other botanical, an amino acid, a dietary substance for use to supplement the diet by increasing the total daily intake, or a concentrate, metabolite, constituent, extract or combinations of these ingredients."

plements can produce negative effects if ingested at improper doses, and some are sold as actual treatments for cancer.

In the absence of government permission to evaluate or regulate the safety or quality of supplements (see Chapter 1), some in the health food industry in conjunction with consumer advocate organizations have stepped in to self-regulate. ConsumerLab.com and the United States Pharmacopeia Dietary Supplement Verification Program are independent groups that routinely evaluate products submitted by manufacturers to ensure that they meet the minimum quality standards. Products that pass all tests are permitted to bear a seal of approval certifying that the product contains the amount specified on the label, has proper bioavailability, and was screened for harmful contaminants.

ConsumerLabs also publishes reports comparing products from different manufacturers. Consumers can use this as a guide to quality products, but neither group evaluates the efficacy of supplements or interactions between supplements and prescription drugs (see Chapter 4), and the submission of products for review is voluntary. Patients should be advised to talk with their physicians or pharmacists before using supplements.

ANTIOXIDANTS

Antioxidants prevent the oxidation of other chemicals and protect the body against damage caused by free radicals, unstable molecules with unpaired electrons generated through metabolism at a cellular level. They react with surrounding compounds causing damage at the level of deoxyribonucleic acid (DNA) and are partially responsible for mutations and carcinogenesis, an effect that can be reversed with antioxidants. Vitamins and supplements such as alpha-lipoic acid, beta-carotene, coenzymeQ10 (ubiquinone), lutein, lycopene, melatonin, N-acetylcysteine, quercetin, selenium, zinc, and vitamins A, C, and E are known to have antioxidant properties and have been used for cancer prevention.

Fruits and vegetables high in antioxidants are known to lower the incidence of certain cancers. Epidemiologic studies show that selenium and vitamin E can reduce the risk of prostate cancer. On the other hand, a major randomized trial of smokers found that beta-carotene supplements, contrary to expectations, increased the risk

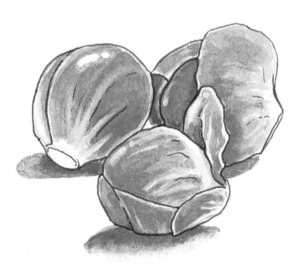

Figure 6-1 Alpha lipoic acid is an essential cofactor and acts as an antioxidant. Food sources include Brussels sprouts, spinach, broccoli, tomato, peas, and rice bran.

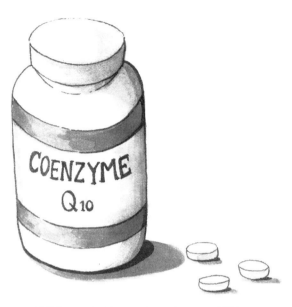

Figure 6-2 Coenzyme Q10 has antioxidant and membrane stabilizing properties.

of lung cancer. It appears to be safer and in all likelihood more beneficial to forego supplements and obtain beta-carotene directly from diet.

Cancer patients use antioxidant supplements to protect against the toxic effects of chemotherapy or to enhance the therapeutic effects of cancer treatment. Whether cancer patients should use antioxidant supplements is still unclear. The use of antioxidants during cancer treatment is complex. Although many believe that chemotherapy and radiotherapy lower the patient's antioxidant status, some studies find no significant change in levels of antioxidants, such as selenium and vitamins C and E, following chemotherapy.

Another concern is whether antioxidant supplements may negatively affect cancer therapies. Radiation therapy and some chemotherapeutic agents, such as anthracycline, platinum compounds, and alkylating agents, rely on the generation of free radicals for their cytotoxic effects. One school of thought maintains that high doses of select antioxidants can protect healthy cells from the damaging effects of chemotherapy and radiation therapy. In fact, prescription drugs such as dexrazoxane are used to reduce the toxicity of chemotherapy because of their antioxidant effects.

Studies also show that high doses of some antioxidants may have direct cytotoxic effects, suggesting that antioxidants may enhance the effect of some therapies. Antioxidants such as vitamins A, C, and E and melatonin can increase the effects of radiation. Studies of the use of antioxidants with chemotherapy produce mixed results, with some showing improved response for certain chemotherapy agents. Most investigations, however, were in vitro and animal studies. Definitive evidence from clinical trials is yet to come.

The opposing school holds that while antioxidants protect healthy cells from free radical damage, they may also protect cancer cells from cytotoxic effects. In vitro studies demonstrate that tumor cells use antioxidants such as vitamin C more efficiently than do normal cells. High levels of antioxidants theoretically may render cancer treatments less effective. For example, beta-carotene reduces the

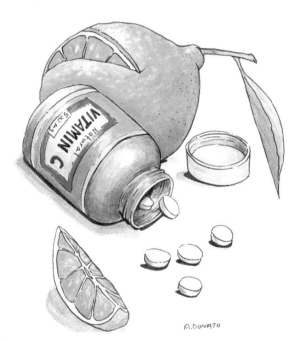

A.DONATO

Figure 6-3 Vitamin C is necessary for a variety of physiologic functions.

effects of 5-fluorouracil (5-FU) in certain cell lines, while vitamin C enhances the resistance of doxorubicin in breast cancer cell lines. These results have not been proven in clinical trials.

The subject of antioxidants in cancer treatment has caused much confusion and remains unresolved. Until more evidence is available indicating otherwise, patients should be advised to avoid large doses of antioxidant supplements during chemotherapy or radiotherapy. A standard multivitamin and antioxidants obtained from dietary sources is optimal at this time. Mainstream nutritionists and physicians rarely recommend high doses of vitamins unless the patient has signs and symptoms of deficiency. However, individuals under metabolic stress or cancer patients unable to maintain good nutrition may benefit from a daily USDA-level multivitamin or mineral supplement.

Some clinicians question whether some of the recommended daily allowance (RDA) recommendations are adequate for cancer prevention or whether additional supplementation may provide useful benefit. The Selenium and Vitamin E Cancer Prevention Trial (SELECT), a prospective clinical trial in which supplemental doses of vitamin E (400 IU) and selenium (200 µg) will be evaluated for their potential to prevent prostate cancer. Studies like these hope to answer the question of whether micronutrient supplements in excess of the RDA offer extra protection against disease.

SOY

Soy contains phytoestrogen (plant-based) isoflavones, which produce estrogenic as well as antiestrogenic effects in laboratory studies. Soy appears to have some preventive effect against breast cancer, but only in women who consumed it around puberty or in large amounts. Following a diagnosis of estrogen-receptor–positive breast cancer, the use of soy products and soy supplements is not advised as these products may stimulate the proliferation of breast lobular epithelium (see Chapter 11). The same concerns pertain to flaxseed, which may have estrogenic effects.

SUPPLEMENTS WITH POTENTIAL ANTICANCER PROPERTIES

Alpha-Lipoic Acid

Alpha-lipoic acid is an endogenous cofactor found in all eukaryotic and prokaryotic cells and obtained from diet. It is essential in the production of energy and acts as a potent antioxidant by functioning as a lipophilic free radical scavenger. Dihydrolipoic acid (DHLA), a reduced form of lipoic acid, has more potent antioxidant effects. It can assist in repairing oxidative damage and regenerate endogenous antioxidants such as vitamins C and E and glutathione. Alpha-lipoic acid causes cell cycle arrest in G0/G1, resulting in cell death in some tumor cell lines. Although it is nontoxic, the antioxidant activity of alpha-lipoic acid may antagonize the effects of chemotherapy and radiation therapy. It should be used with caution.

Beta-Carotone

A natural pigment synthesized by plants. Beta-carotene supplements are used as antioxidants and immunostimulants and to prevent or treat cancer, human immunodeficiency virus (HIV), heart disease, and leukoplakia. Proposed mechanisms of action for cancer prevention include inhibition of cancer growth, induction of differentiation by modulation of cell cycle regulatory proteins, alterations in insulin-like growth factor-1, prevention of oxidative DNA damage, and possible enhancement of carcinogen metabolizing enzymes. Beta-carotene may enhance macrophage function, NK-cell cytotoxicity and increase T-helper lymphocytes. A meta-analysis of eight randomized trials demonstrated a small but significant increase in all-cause mortality and cardiovascular death in patients using beta-carotene compared with placebo. Beta-carotene supplementation is not advised.

D-Limonene

Derived from the peels of citrus fruits, D-Limonene is used as a supplement to prevent and treat cancer. D-Limonene and its metabolites, perillic acid, dihydroperillic acid, uroterpenol, and limonene1,2-diol, may inhibit tumor growth via inhibition of p21-dependent signaling. D-Limonene metabolites also cause G1 cell cycle arrest, inhibit posttranslational modification of signal transduction proteins, and cause differential expression of cell cycle- and apoptosis-related genes. Animal studies show activity of D-limonene against pancreatic, stomach, colon, skin, and liver cancers. Data also indicate that this substance slows the promotion or progression stage of carcinogen-induced tumors in rats. Further research will determine if D-Limonene has a role in cancer prevention or treatment.

Flaxseed

Derived from the seeds of a slender annual plant, flaxseed is also known as linseed. Traditionally used to treat coughs, colds, constipation, and urinary tract infections, it also is used as a topical demulcent and emollient. Flaxseed is a concentrated source of omega-3 fatty acids and phytoestrogenic lignans with chemoprotective effects. It may also benefit patients with lupus nephritis. Animal studies suggest that flaxseed may inhibit the growth and metastasis of human melanoma and breast and prostate cancers. Caution is advised for patients with estrogen-receptor–positive breast cancer, as flaxseed contains phytoestrogens. Flaxseed lowered prostate cancer biomarkers in a pilot study but did not influence oral mucous membrane flora in patients radiated for head and neck cancer. Side effects of flaxseed supplementation are minor gastrointestinal distress, but cases of anaphylaxis and immunologically positive antigen response were reported as well. Ingestion of flaxseed may interfere with radiology procedures.

Folic Acid

A water-soluble vitamin of the vitamin B complex, folic acid, or folate, reduces the risk of neural tube defects and is an essential supplement during pregnancy. Higher levels of folic acid reduce risk for cancers of the breast, pancreas, and colon. Folic acid reduces homocysteine levels and blood pressure in smokers. Studies on the risk of stroke yield mixed results. The bioavailability of folate tends to be greater from supplements than from natural food sources, and some benefits of folate are increased when taken with other vitamins. Folic acid and methotrexate are mutually antagonistic. Folic acid may reduce the efficacy of methotrexate in the treatment of acute lymphoblastic leukemia.

Lycopene

Lycopene, a carotenoid with antioxidant activity, is a pigment synthesized by plants and microorganisms. Epidemiologic studies suggest an inverse relationship between lycopene consumption and risk of cancer, particularly lung, prostrate, and stomach cancers. Proposed mechanisms of action in prevention include inhibition of cancer growth, induction of differentiation by modulation of cell cycle regulatory proteins, alterations in insulin-like growth factor-1, prevention of oxidative DNA damage, and possible enhancement of carcinogen-metabolizing enzymes. Other possible actions for all carotenoids include immunoenhancement, inhibition of mutagenesis and transformation, and inhibition of premalignant lesions. Small clinical trials show possible benefit in cancer, but no optimal dosage has been established and larger clinical trials are needed.

Melatonin

Melatonin is a hormonal supplement primarily of synthetic origin but occasionally derived from animal sources. Patients use melatonin to treat insomnia, jet lag, and cancer. Melatonin is produced endogenously in the pineal gland. Exogenous melatonin is absorbed poorly following oral administration and is metabolized rapidly by the liver. Melatonin is thought to control the circadian pacemaker and promote sleep. Melatonin appears to be a potent free radical scavenger. It demonstrates antiproliferative effects on cancer cell lines both in vitro and in animal models. Clinical trials evaluating melatonin as monotherapy and in combination with other agents in patients with solid tumors suggest improvements in quality of life. It also increases survival time and tumor response in patients treated with tamoxifen, cisplatin, and etopside and in patients with brain glioblastomas undergoing radiotherapy. Reported adverse effects include drowsiness, headache, hypothermia, pruritus, abdominal cramps, and tachycardia. Melatonin may interact with nifedipine, resulting in elevated blood pressure and heart rate.

N-Acetylcysteine

N-acetylcysteine (NAC) is an endogenous antioxidant and precursor to intracellular glutathione. NAC is approved as a mucolytic agent for treatment of respiratory diseases and as an antidote to acetaminophen poisoning. NAC has antioxidant, nucleophilic, mucolytic, and possibly chemopreventive properties. In animal models, NAC inhibits a variety of mutagen- and carcinogen-induced cancer biomarkers, interferes with the promotion phase of multi-stage carcinogenesis, and decreases the incidence of carcinogen-induced tumors of lung, colon, and bladder. This activity may be owing to its ability to enhance glutathione S-transferases, glutathione peroxidase, glutathione reductase, and nicotinamide adenine dinucleotide (NADH)- and NADPH-quinone reductase. Animal studies suggest anticarcinogenic, antimetastatic, and antiangiogenic activity. Studies in smokers and patients with history of adenomatous colonic polyps show inhibition of cancer biomarker development. However, NAC did not inhibit formation of secondary head and neck or lung tumors. Human studies evaluating the role of NAC in preventing chemotherapy- or radiotherapy-induced toxicities are inconclusive.

Quercetin

Quercetin is a flavonoid readily available in dietary plants such as tea, onion, apple, and buckwheat. It is thought to have antioxidant activity due to the reactivity of its phenolic group, which reacts with free radicals to form the more stable phenoxy radicals. Quercetin is thought to have anti-inflammatory and antiallergy properties. The proposed mechanism of action is the inhibition of lipoxygenase and cyclooxygenase, resulting in reduced production of inflammatory mediators (eg, leukotrienes and histamine). Quercetin appears to inhibit cyclooxygenase to a greater degree than does lipoxygenase. Proposed anticancer mechanisms of action include downregulation of mutant p53 proteins; G1 phase arrest; tyrosine kinase inhibition; estrogen receptor binding; inhibition of heat shock proteins; and ras-protein expression inhibition. Presently, considerable in vitro data support the concept of quercetin as an anticancer compound, but there are few clinical studies and results are mixed.

Selenium

Selenium is an essential trace element required by the glutathione–peroxidase pathway. It supports the actions of other antioxidants and the reduction of vitamin C. Clinical studies evaluating the role of selenium in cancer prevention produced intriguing results. The ongoing SELECT study, conducted by the Southwest Oncology

Group, aims to reveal the effects of selenium on cancer. Selenium effectively reduces therapy-related lymphedema. Animal studies suggest it can decrease the nephrotoxic effect of cisplatin while increasing its antitumor activity. Adverse effects from selenium usually are gastric in nature, although chronic selenosis can occur with doses greater than 1000 µg/day. This toxicity is characterized by muscle weakness, fatigue, peripheral neuropathy, skin rash, nail and hair changes, irritability, and possibly hepatic necrosis. Long-term use of selenium may increase the risk of certain types of skin cancer.

Ubiquinone

Patients use this supplement to treat cancer, congestive heart failure, arrhythmias, Parkinson's disease, and hypertension and to prevent anthracycline cardiomyopathy. Ubiquinone, commonly known as coenzyme Q_{10} is essential for the production of adenosine triphosphate. It also has antioxidant properties. Ubiquinone is structurally similar to vitamin K and therefore may interact with warfarin. It may antagonize the effects of chemotherapy via antioxidant activity.

Vitamin C

Vitamin C is a water-soluble vitamin necessary for a variety of physiologic functions. Clinical studies suggest no survival advantage or antineoplastic activity with vitamin C. In addition, in vitro and animal studies suggest that cancer cells preferentially uptake vitamin C, suggesting that high-dose supplementation may have negative effects for cancer patients. In animal and in vitro studies, vitamin C can decrease the toxicity as well as the efficacy of doxorubicin. Some studies show that vitamin C may potentiate the effects of radiotherapy. Potential adverse effects are gastrointestinal in nature, although hypoglycemia and hypotension are documented for doses greater than 1 g/day. Patients with a history of oxalate kidney stones, renal insufficiency, glucose-6-phosphate dehydrogenase (G6PDH) deficiency, or hematochromatosis should use vitamin C with caution.

Vitamin E

Derived from plant oils and foods, including wheat germ, eggs, green leafy vegetables, and whole grains, vitamin E (d-α-tocopherol) acts as an antioxidant. Its main function is to prevent propagation of free radicals by acting as a peroxyl radical scavenger and protecting polyunsaturated fatty acids within membrane phospholipids and in plasma lipoproteins. It reportedly inhibits protein kinase C activity, which is involved in cell proliferation and differentiation in smooth muscle cells, human platelets, and monocytes. Vitamin E enrichment of endothelial cells downregulates the expression of intercellular adhesion molecule (ICAM-1) and vascular cell adhesion molecule-1 (VCAM-1), decreasing the adhesion of blood cell components to the endothelium. It also upregulates the expression of cytosolic phospholipase A2 and cyclooxegenase-1, which releases prostacyclin, a potent vasodilator and inhibitor of platelet aggregation in humans. Studies evaluating vitamin E supplementation suggest it may reduce the risk of some cancers and the incidence of cisplatin-induced neurotoxicity. Studies of effects on radiation therapy yield mixed results. A clinical trial found that 800 IU of vitamin E daily reduced hot flashes in breast cancer survivors. There are no significant adverse effects, although toxicity may occur with chronic doses greater than 800 IU. A recent meta-analysis suggests a daily dose of more than 400 IU vitamin E may increase all-cause mortality. Theoretically, vitamin E may enhance the activity of warfarin, but data are inconsistent.

CONCLUSION

Many supplements are promoted as viable cancer treatments or cancer cures. Such uses are dangerous, but patients often are attracted to glowing albeit invalid promotional claims; these are discussed in Chapter 19.

READINGS AND RESOURCES

1. Agus DB, Vera JC, Golde DW. Stromal cell oxidation: a mechanism by which tumors obtain vitamin C. Cancer Res 1999;59:4555–8.
2. Cassileth BR, Lucarelli C. Herb-drug interactions in oncology. Hamilton (ON): BC Decker, Inc; 2003.
3. Conklin KA. Dietary antioxidants during cancer chemotherapy: impact on chemotherapeutic effectiveness and development of side effects. Nutr Cancer 2000;37:1–18.
4. Labriola D, Livingston R. Possible interactions between dietary antioxidants and chemotherapy. Oncology (Huntington) 1999;13:1003–8.
5. Ladas EJ, Jacobson JS, Kennedy DD, et al. Antioxidants and cancer therapy: a systematic review. J Clin Oncol 2004;22:517–28.
6. National Cancer Institute. Nutrition in cancer care. Available at:

http://www.cancer.gov/cancertopics/pdq/supportivecare/nutrition/HealthProf essional (accessed March 10, 2004).

7. Prasad KN, Cole WC, Kumar B, et al. Scientific rationale for using high-dose multiple micronutrients as an adjunct to standard and experimental cancer therapies. J Amer Coll Nutr 2001;20(Suppl 5):450S–463S.

8. Miller ER, et al. Meta-analysis: high-dosage vitamin E supplementation may increase all-cause mortality. Ann Intern Med. 2005 Jan 4;142(1):37-46.

9. Seifried HE, Anderson DE, Sorkin BC, Costello RB. Free radicals: The pros and cons of antioxidants. Executive Summary Report of the June 26-27 NIH conference on "Free Radicals: The pros and cons of antioxidants. J Nutr 134:3143-3163S.

7

Mind–Body Therapies

Cognitive behavior therapy, biofeedback, guided imagery, hypnosis, meditation, and relaxation approaches comprise mind–body therapies. All have a role in cancer care. Their value lies not only in their effectiveness in providing symptom relief, but also in the fact that these are pleasant, noninvasive interventions from among which patients can select according to their preference and use to help manage their own clinical care.

In a national survey, 19% of adults in the United States had used at least one mind–body therapy in the previous year. A meta-analysis of 116 studies showed that mind–body therapies were beneficial in treating anxiety, depression, mood disturbance, and coping in cancer patients. Research evaluating specific mind–body interventions is reviewed below.

RELAXATION TECHNIQUES

Relaxation training involving progressive muscle relaxation has been studied in randomized controlled trials, which demonstrate that it significantly ameliorates anxiety and distress and is particularly effective when combined with imagery. A randomized study of relaxation therapy versus alprazolam showed that both significantly decreased anxiety and depression, although the effect of alprazolam was slightly faster in anxiety and stronger on depressive symptoms. Progressive relaxation achieves similar effects without side effects and at less cost.

A randomized trial of 82 radiation therapy patients found significant reductions in tension, depression, anger, and fatigue in those who received relaxation training or imagery. Cardiac studies find similar results. However, research shows that relaxation techniques themselves induce anxiety in 17 to 31%, most often because of patients' intrusive thoughts, fear of losing control, and restlessness. Other mind–body interventions may be more appropriate for some cancer patients.

HYPNOSIS

Hypnosis reduces anxiety and distress. It has also been studied extensively and found effective for a wide range of symptoms, including acute and chronic pain, panic, phobias, pediatric emergencies, surgery, burns, posttraumatic stress disorder (PTSD), irritable bowel syndrome (IBS), allergies, certain skin conditions, and unwanted habit control. Nausea and vomiting prevention using presurgical hypnosis for 50 breast surgery patients in a randomized controlled trial revealed 29% less vomiting and less nausea in the hypnosis group over the standard-care control group.

In a recent study, 204 IBS patients attended 12 one-hour hypnotherapy sessions. Seventy-one percent reported improvements after the course, and 81% of those maintained the improvements 5 years later. Hypnosis effectively manages pain associated with limb surgery and limb rehabilitation. In 60 hand surgery patients, the hypnosis group experienced significantly less pain and anxiety than did those randomized to standard care. Surgeons' rating of patient progress was higher for the hypnosis patients, and fewer medical complications occurred in the hypnosis group. Hypnosis is also an effective intervention for the relief of phantom pain.

Hypnosis has a long and useful history in pain management. It reduces postoperative use of pain medication and appears to be effective across many surgical procedures. Meta-analyses of hypnosis across surgical populations found positive effects in 89% of patients, with significant benefits in both subjective pain indicators and objective outcomes including pain medication, physiologic indicators, recovery time, and treatment time. In a procedural study, 30 patients scheduled for interventional radiology procedures were randomized to hypnosis or standard care. The hypnosis group reported less pain and exhibited more stable oxygen saturation and hemodynamics. Recent perioperative trials demonstrate broad benefits from adjunctive hypnosis, including reduced pre- and postsurgical anxiety and depression, fewer postsurgery complications, more stable vital signs perioperatively, faster healing, less postoperative pain medication use, and increased patient and surgeon satisfaction with the procedures.

Research shows that hypnosis does not work by eliciting endorphin release. Rather, hypnotic suggestion for analgesia involves reduction in spinal cord antinociceptive mechanisms, prevention of awareness of pain once nociception has reached higher centers via brain mechanisms, and reduction of affect dimensions, possibly through reinterpretation of meanings associated with the painful sensations.

Pain and anxiety frequently are studied together as their outcomes typically are linked. In a randomized control study, 60 elective surgery patients were assigned to hypnosis or emotional support. The hypnotherapy group reported significantly less peri- and postoperative pain and anxiety, and this was confirmed by independent psychologist observers. Vital signs were significantly more stable in the hypnosis group and pain medications were reduced.

In a randomized trial, 241 percutaneous vascular and renal procedure patients were randomized to standard care, standard care plus hypnosis, or standard care plus structured attention. The hypnosis group fared significantly better in terms of anxiety, drug use, hemodynamic stability, and procedure time. A study of perioperative anxiety in hypnosis patients compared with standard control subjects showed that anxiety decreased more sharply in hypnosis patients than in control subjects. Hypnosis is cost-effective considering improved recovery time and decreased pain medication use. In a study of outpatient interventional radiologic procedures, costs were reduced by almost 53% by hypnosis versus standard pharmacologic sedation.

Hypnosis is especially effective with children. Fifty-four pediatric cancer patients were randomly assigned to hypnosis, nonhypnotic distraction and relaxation, or attention control. Children in the hypnosis group reported the greatest reduction in anticipatory and postchemotherapy nausea and vomiting. Symptoms in the cognitive distraction and relaxation intervention did not change substantively, and symptoms in the attention control group consistently worsened over time. Children undergoing multiple painful procedures such as bone marrow aspiration or lumbar puncture were evaluated before and after mind–body therapy. Hypnosis significantly reduced pain and anxiety. Nonhypnotic behavior techniques produced smaller but still significant benefits.

Contrary to popular belief, hypnosis is effective for most people, with recent research finding less than 10 to 15% of the population unresponsive to it. Trance, or hypnotic state, uses imagination and imagery, but it taps neurologic brain centers other than those evoked

Hypnosis was endorsed by the British Medical Society in 1955 and by the American Medical Association in 1958. The US National Institutes of Health in 1996 cited hypnosis as an effective adjunct in alleviating cancer pain.

by daydreaming or imagination. Instead, it is closely related to a dissociated level of awareness. In a study of 95 randomly assigned dental patients, hypnotic treatment alone was 99% efficacious in providing analgesia for procedural comfort. Because there is little in the way of risk with hypnosis (see below for cautions), the risk-benefit ratio is favorable.

CONTRAINDICATIONS AND CAUTIONS

As in any clinical specialty, it is important to use or refer patients to properly trained and credentialed clinicians. Negative effects from hypnosis are minimal and unusual, with less than 5 to 31% reporting mild dizziness, nausea, or headache. However, such occurrences were attributable to practitioner failure to properly bring patients out of trance. Caution is necessary with high-risk mental health populations, including patients vulnerable to psychotic decompensation, paranoid ideation, unstable dissociation, and borderline character structure. However, problems are more likely to occur with intense application of hypnosis in psychotherapeutic settings, as opposed to adjunctive medical symptom management. Research shows that hypnosis is most effective for symptoms of physiologic origin. Psychological problems should be identified and managed first and separately. Some patients use distress for secondary gain, for example, to obtain family support or attention.

GUIDED IMAGERY AND VISUALIZATION

Guided imagery may be considered a lighter form of hypnosis. It is a simple and powerful technique that directs imagination and attention in ways that produce symptom relief. Often termed "visualization" or "mental imagery," guided imagery lowers blood pressure and produces other physiologic benefits, including decreased heart rate. Imagery also can relieve pain and anxiety. A study of 93 women with locally advanced breast cancer compared standard treatment with versus without relaxation training and imagery during chemotherapy. Women in the experimental group reported increased relaxation and better quality of life during treatment. Similarly, guided imagery increased patient comfort in a randomized trial of 53 breast cancer patients receiving radiation therapy.

A review of 67 published studies indicates that relaxation, imagery, and suggestion impact cancer-related pain. In a trial of 110 breast cancer patients undergoing autologous bone marrow transplantation, patients were randomized to standard care versus education, cognitive restructuring, and relaxation with guided imagery. The experimental group experienced significantly reduced nausea and anxiety.

MEDITATION

The role of meditation in health care has been studied scientifically in the West throughout the last two decades. Its value in the management of physiologic symptoms such as chronic pain, hypertension, and symptoms associated with heart disease and cancer are well documented. Regular meditation also decreases generalized anxiety, wards off bouts of chronic depression, and enables patients to cope more effectively.

The Mindfulness-Based Stress Reduction clinic at the University of Massachusetts Medical Center was the first Western medical facility to research and institutionalize the benefits of meditation and is one of the few mind–body programs authorized to receive third-party reimbursement. The program has trained more than 5,000 health care professionals worldwide in the past 20 years to use meditation in the management of stress and pain.

In a randomized controlled study, meditation achieved significantly greater physical relaxation and better mood when compared with a progressive muscle relaxation group. In another study, 59 breast and prostate cancer patients pursued an 8-week meditation and relaxation training program. Significant improvements occurred in overall quality of life, symptoms of stress, and sleep quality.

A recent randomized clinical trial of 39 patients with lymphoma demonstrated that yoga with controlled breathing and visualization significantly reduced sleep disturbance compared with wait-list control subjects. A meta-analysis of 59 studies showed improved sleep induction and maintenance with psychological interventions, including meditation, biofeedback, and muscle relaxation. Some studies suggest that, while pharmaceuticals produce a rapid response, behavioral therapies such as meditation and imagery help maintain long-term improvement in sleep quality.

Physiologic Change

The effects of meditation on mood and the brain have been studied with functional magnetic resonance imaging (MRI) techniques at the University of Wisconsin and elsewhere. Brain activity in the frontal cortex during meditation is observed to shift from a baseline right orientation (anxious, angry, depressed) to a baseline left orientation (enthusiastic, relaxed, happy).

With long-term use (more than 1 year) antiaddictive effects become apparent. A recent study showed that immune functioning is higher in meditators compared with nonmeditators. Numerous studies demonstrate that stress-related illnesses such as hypertension, high blood pressure associated with bronchial asthma, insomnia, and premature ventricular contractions associated with heart disease respond to meditation, often enabling significant reductions in hypertensive medications.

Meditation is simple, but its benefits require daily practice. As little as 10 minutes once or twice a day can effect dramatic reductions in pain, positive symptom management, increased calm, and alleviated anxiety and stress. However, its rewards are fleeting when practice is stopped.

BIOFEEDBACK

Biofeedback is effective for high blood pressure, chronic pain, migraine headaches, alcoholism, drug abuse, and anxiety. It is used to facilitate relaxation in treating muscle injury, chronic muscle pain, and stiffness. Electrodermal activity measurements and finger pulse feedback are used in the treatment of anxiety as well as hypertension and cardiac arrhythmias. Respiration feedback can help alleviate asthma, hyperventilation, and anxiety.

Biofeedback has helped overcome urinary incontinence by developing more effective control of bladder muscles. A recent randomized clinical trial involving 42 patients with urinary incontinence following radical prostatectomy showed that biofeedback was effective in early management. It can also assist the retraining of body muscles after accident or surgery and help train new muscles to take over the function of those that are irreparably damaged. A meta-analysis showed a pooled odds ratio of 2:1 favoring the addition of biofeedback to pelvic floor muscle exercises versus pelvic floor exercises alone, but this was not supported by a larger randomized trial.

Biofeedback research in oncology has produced mixed results. A study of 81 cancer patients randomized to standard care, relaxation training, or biofeedback training assessed nausea, anxiety, and physiological arousal over the course of five consecutive chemotherapy treatments. Relaxation patients had decreased nausea and anxiety during chemotherapy. Biofeedback had no effect on chemotherapy side effects. Such findings suggest that relaxation training may reduce the adverse consequences of chemotherapy but that the positive effects for biofeedback may be a result of the relaxation component rather than the biofeedback alone.

MIND–BODY THERAPIES AND END-OF-LIFE CARE

Many of the symptoms addressed in this chapter are even more prevalent during end-of-life cancer care, and mind–body therapies are especially useful in managing terminal illness. They can relieve symptoms without oversedation, allowing patients and families valuable and viable time together. Family caregivers can contribute to the patient's comfort using guided imagery and relaxation techniques. This has the added advantage of giving caregivers a sense of control and of contributing to the patient's well-being.

READINGS AND RESOURCES

1. Carlson LE, Ursuliak Z, Goodey E, et al. The effects of a mindfulness meditation-based stress reduction program on mood and symptoms of stress in cancer outpatients: 6-month follow-up. Support Care Cancer 2001;9:112–23.
2. Davidson RJ, Kabat-Zinn J, Schumacher J, et al. Alterations in brain and immune function produced by mindfulness meditation. Psychosom Med 2003;65:564–70.

3. Kabat-Zinn J, Massion AO, Herbert JR, Rosenbaum E. Meditation. In: Holland J, editor. Psycho-oncology. Oxford: Oxford University Press;1998. p 767–79.

4. Montgomery GH, David D, Winkel G, et al. The effectiveness of adjunctive hypnosis with surgical patients: a meta-analysis. Anesth Analg 2002;94:1639–45.

5 National Institutes of Health Technology Assessment panel. Integration of behavioral and relaxation approaches into the treatment of chronic pain and insomnia. NIH Technology Assessment Conference Statement. 1995;Oct 16–18:1–34. Available at: http://consensus.nih.gov/ta/017/017_statement.htm (accessed March 10, 2005).

8

Acupuncture

Acupuncture, a treatment modality used initially in traditional Chinese medicine (see Chapter 2) and increasingly accepted today in the West involves the stimulation of one or more predetermined points on the body with needles, heat, pressure, or electricity for therapeutic effect.

The Word Health Organization supports the practice of acupuncture as an effective intervention for the following problems:
- Adverse reactions to radiotherapy and chemotherapy
- Depression (including depressive neurosis and depression following stroke)
- Facial pain (including craniomandibular disorders)
- Headache
- Leukopenia
- Lower back pain
- Nausea and vomiting
- Neck pain
- Postoperative pain

In the United States, acupuncture has been practiced in immigrant Chinese communities for many decades, but only in recent years has it become more broadly accepted as a viable treatment option. A recent Centers for Disease Control and Prevention report indicates that more than 8 million Americans use acupuncture for various ailments. A 1997 National Institutes of Health Consensus Conference concluded that acupuncture effectively treats lower back pain, osteoarthritis, and nausea. Since that time, however, research has confirmed its utility in treating many additional symptoms. This is particularly relevant with regard to the care of cancer patients, as many serious symptoms experienced by these patients are not well managed with mainstream conventional therapies.

The Food and Drug Administration categorizes acupuncture needles as medical devices and restricts their use to qualified practitioners. Acupuncturists in the United States use sterile, disposable, filiform needles, typically made of stainless steel and commonly packed in a guide tube to assist swift insertion (Figure 8-1). The insertion of acupuncture needles causes minimal or no pain and much less tissue injury than occurs with phlebotomy or parenteral injections.

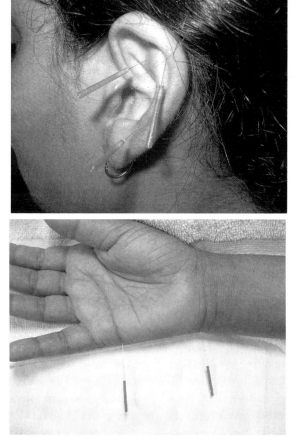

Figure 8-1 Acupuncture is safe and can be used to control many symptoms associated with cancer and cancer treatment.

- There are approximately 50 acupuncture training programs in the United States, most requiring more than 3 years of full-time postgraduate training. National certification is governed by the National Certification Commission for Acupuncture and Oriental Medicine (NCCAOM) in Washington, DC, which has certified over 9,000 practitioners in 47 states and 18 foreign countries.
- Some states allow licensed physicians and dentists to practice medical acupuncture following 200 to 300 hours of training. The American Academy of Medical Acupuncture certifies eligible physician-acupuncturists.

MECHANISMS OF ACTION

Acupuncture is an intrinsic component of traditional Chinese medicine theory (see Chapter 2), which is based on the ancient theory of balance between yin and yang and the flow of Qi (energy) along hypothesized channels (meridians) in the body. Acupuncture points are located at specific points along the channels. The flow of Qi, and therefore health, was thought to be regulated by the needling of these points.

Many health professionals who practice acupuncture, especially those in the United States, dispense with such traditional theory. The anatomic structures representing meridians remain elusive to this date. However, some acupuncture points coincide with trigger points that are sensitive to pressure, indicating enriched enervation at the anatomic location. Stimulation of certain acupuncture points does produce measurable physiologic change.

Animal studies in the early 1970s demonstrated that acupuncture-induced analgesia can be blocked by naloxone, a narcotic antagonist. More recently, mice deficient in opiate receptors were shown to be refractory to acupuncture, and levels of β-endorphin in human cerebrospinal fluid were found to increase following acupuncture, suggesting that acupuncture stimulates their release. Acupuncture also was shown to regulate the production of serotonin and is known to stimulate A delta fibers that enter the dorsal horn of the spinal cord. This mediates segmental inhibition of pain impulses carried in the slower unmyelinated C fibers and, through connections in the midbrain, enhances inhibition of descending C fiber pain impulses at other levels of the spinal cord. This provides one explanation of how acupuncture produces effects distant from needling points.

Stimulation of the auricular LU 1 point can elevate parasympathetic function, and stimulation of the LI 4 point elevates both sympathetic and parasympathetic tone. These effects, observed when heart rate variability is used as a measure of sympathetic and parasympathetic function, may help explain why acupuncture treats symptoms such as shortness of breath, diarrhea, and xerostomia.

Functional magnetic resonance imaging (fMRI) provides a new tool with which to study the neurologic effects of acupuncture treatment. It has enabled documentation of activity in areas of the brain associated with acupuncture-stimulated functions or organs. Recent studies using fMRI technology have shed light on the specific nervous pathways possibly involved in acupuncture. Activation of neuronal activity has been observed in the hypothalamus and nucleus accumbens, and deactivation in the anterior cingulate cortex, amygdala, and hippocampus during true acupuncture. These changes are not found in control stimulations, which are associated only with changes in the sensory cortex.

Deactivation of amygdala and hippocampus also have been reported in electroacupuncture. In addition, the degree of signal intensity appears to correlate with analgesic effect. Because many of these areas of the brain are involved in the cognitive-affective aspects of pain perception (see Chapter 15), these findings suggest that acupuncture may reduce the sensation of pain also by altering pain perception.

CLINICAL ASSESSMENT AND TREATMENT PLAN

Traditionally trained acupuncturists examine the tongue and palpate the pulse to assess the patient's condition, while Western-trained medical practitioners usually perform standard physical examinations. Following determination of a treatment plan for problems identified, needles are inserted into relevant acupuncture points and retained for 20 to 30 minutes. Acupuncture points usually are located in depressions between joints, muscle fascia, or sensitive points along hypothesized channels.

Some patients may feel a minor pinch as needles puncture the skin, but most report no pain or discomfort. To enhance treatment effects, acupuncturists may manually manipulate the needles or connect the their free ends to the wires of a low-voltage electrostimulation device. Occasionally, moxibustion (see below) may be applied to achieve the same goal.

TYPES OF NEEDLES

Intradermal Needles

Intradermal needles are extremely fine, semipermanent needles that may be left in place for 1 week or more to provide continuous stimulation over longer periods of time. Some are straight wheat-grain–type needles with a small looped handle. They are inserted transversely a few millimeters into the point. Also called tack-needles or studs, intradermal needles, pictured below (Figure 8-2), are short (1–2 mm long) needles embedded in hypoallergenic adhesive tape. They are similar in appearance to a miniature thumbtack. Inserted perpendicularly, they are then covered with Tegaderm to protect against infection.

These in-dwelling needles hold great promise in facilitating acupuncture for patients who cannot return often to receive traditional acupuncture. The inconvenience and expense of frequent visits

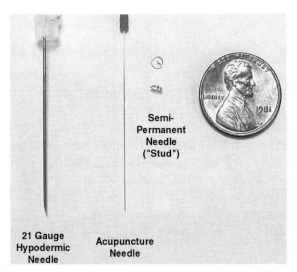

Figure 8-2 Acupuncture uses very fine, filiform, disposable needles.

to acupuncturists represent the primary barrier to use of acupuncture treatment in the West.

Ear Seeds

Ear seeds are tiny, sesame seed–sized magnetized metallic pellets or seeds of *Vaccaria segetalis*, an herb commonly used in Chinese medicine. These are taped on acupuncture points and may be stimulated by the patient to enhance their effect.

AURICULAR ACUPUNCTURE

This approach uses the outer ear as a microsystem of the entire body. Needles or seeds are strategically placed to relieve symptoms. Auricular acupuncture can be used alone or with body points.

INCREASING THE STIMULATION OF ACUPUNCTURE NEEDLES

- Electroacupuncture: Low-voltage electric impulses attached after insertion to the free end of needles are used to provide increased, continuous stimulation. Various frequencies and intensities are applied according to the patient's condition and tolerance. This approach is especially useful for musculoskeletal pain, pruritus, and neuropathy.
- Moxibustion: A method used to stimulate acupuncture points through heat, which is delivered via a burning plug of moxa, a compacted cone of the herb mugwort (artemisia). Moxa may be applied over the acupoints in a pecking motion, or placed on the skin, although this method is discouraged in modern practice.
- Acupressure: Finger, palm, or elbow pressure is applied to increase stimulation of acupoints. Shiatsu is a form of acupressure developed in Japan.

The needling sensation, or "De qi,"—a numbness, pressure, or tingling—may be perceived by the patient during or after insertion of acupuncture needles. This sensation is thought to be associated with the efficacy of acupuncture and is sometimes used to judge whether the needle is inserted at the proper location. Not all patients report this sensation, and some points may be more sensitive than others. In addition to symptom relief, patients often indicate feeling relaxed or energized during and following acupuncture. Follow-up treatments, typically once or twice weekly for several weeks, may be necessary to achieve optimal benefit.

Adverse Effects

When performed by trained practitioners, acupuncture is safe. Studies in Europe and Japan show that less than 0.2% of individuals treated with acupuncture experience adverse effects. The most commonly reported adverse events are failure to remove needles, bleeding, hematoma, dizziness, and pain. In more severe but rare cases, pneumothorax, local infections, and burns caused by moxibustion have been reported.

Even with good aseptic technique, it is prudent not to use acupuncture for patients with neutropenia, thrombocytopenia, or at risk for endocarditis due to heart valve abnormality. Because acupuncture can cause uterine contractions, caution should be exercised in the treatment of pregnant women, with particular acupuncture points contraindicated. Needles should not be placed in the affected limb of patients with lymphedema. Electrical stimulation is contraindicated for patients wearing pacemakers or other electronic medical devices.

INDICATIONS FOR ACUPUNCTURE IN CANCER CARE

Nausea and Vomiting

The pharmacologic treatment of chemotherapy-related nausea and vomiting has improved substantially in recent years, but some patients still experience these symptoms. Acupuncture effectively treats nausea and vomiting. In a review of 19 clinical trials of postoperative vomiting, acupuncture cut the rate of vomiting by half. A randomized trial of 104 breast cancer patients showed that electroacupuncture was more effective than placebo needling and more effective than pharmaceuticals in relieving chemotherapy-induced emesis. Acupuncture may work best against nausea and vomiting when given before chemotherapy, as its benefit seems to last about 8 hours. Acupuncture

> Electroacupuncture was more effective than placebo and pharmaceuticals in relieving chemotherapy-induced emesis.

is especially recommended for poorly controlled acute or subacute nausea in cancer patients.

Wrist bands that stimulate the inner-wrist nausea acupoint with a small electric current have not proved effective, but pressing that point with fingers of the other hand often provides relief.

Chronic Pain

Randomized trials largely support acupuncture for both acute pain, such as in dental surgery, and chronic pain, as with migraine headaches. A randomized, blinded, controlled trial of 90 cancer patients showed that auricular acupuncture reduced their pain. After two courses of treatment, pain intensity decreased 36% from baseline as compared with 2% in placebo control subjects. Several single-arm studies also suggest a benefit for acupuncture in the management of pain associated with metastatic disease. Acupuncture should be considered for patients experiencing chronic cancer pain, particularly if poorly controlled by appropriately titrated medication or if the medication is causing unacceptable adverse effects.

Neuropathy

Long-term sequelae of chemotherapy, radiation therapy, and surgery include difficult-to-manage neuropathic pain (see Chapter 15). Acupuncture appears to ameliorate persistent neuropathic pain following thoracotomy, mastectomy, and radical neck dissection. Chemotherapeutic agents such as taxane or platinum compounds also may cause peripheral neuropathy.

A recent randomized, blinded, controlled trial confirmed the benefits of auricular acupuncture in reducing cancer pain that persisted despite stable analgesic treatment. Ninety patients were randomized to needles placed at correct acupuncture points (treatment group), needles placed at nonacupuncture points, or application of pressure at nonacupuncture points. Pain intensity decreased by 36% two months later in the treatment group, a significant difference compared with the control groups, where little pain reduction occurred. These results are especially important because many patients in this trial had pain that was refractory to conventional treatment.

Xerostomia

Acupuncture appears to be effective in the treatment of xerostomia, especially when applied shortly after radiation therapy damage to the salivary gland. Larger, more definitive randomized trials are underway.

Mood Disturbance

As detailed in Chapter 16, acupuncture can decrease mood disturbance in cancer patients.

READINGS AND RESOURCES

1. American Academy of Medical Acupuncture. http://www.medicalacupuncture.org/index.html (accessed Sept 16, 2004).
2. National Center for Complementary and Alternative Medicine. Acupuncture [research report]. National Center for Complementary and Alternative Medicine. Available at: http://nccam.nih.gov/health/acupuncture/ (accessed Sept 16, 2004).
3. National Institutes of Health. Acupuncture: Consensus Development Conference Statement. National Institutes of Health. November 3–5, 1997. Available at: http://odp.od.nih.gov/consensus/cons/107/107_statement.htm (accessed March 10, 2005).
4. World Health Organization. Acupuncture: Review and Analysis of Reports on Controlled Clinical Trials. World Health Organization; 2002. Available at: http://www.who.int/medicines/library/trm/acupuncture/acupuncture_trials.pdf (accessed Sept 16, 2004).

9

Bodywork

Bodywork includes various forms of self-driven, active exercise as well as passive receipt of interventions such as massage therapy. These noninvasive therapies relieve distress, improve quality of life, and reduce many symptoms associated with cancer and cancer treatment. Complementary therapies involving bodywork, including exercise, tai chi, Qigong, yoga, and massage therapy are described below.

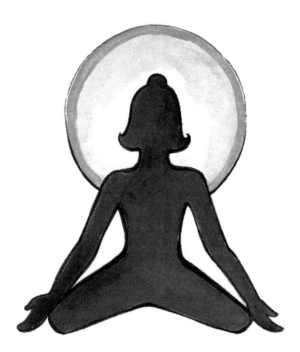

EXERCISE

Fatigue is among the most common and troublesome symptoms that cancer patients experience. Fatigue may be caused or exacerbated by radiotherapy and chemotherapy, medication, tumor-related factors, or stress. Loss of muscle mass is a key factor, eventually leading to impaired physical performance and consequent diminishment of physical and emotional quality of life. A regular exercise program helps patients improve stamina, agility, muscle tone, and flexibility and is now a standard of care for cancer-related fatigue. Relevant research is summarized below; fatigue is discussed in greater detail in Chapter 16.

In a controlled trial in Scotland of 66 men receiving radiotherapy for localized prostate cancer, patients were randomized to moderate-intensity walking for 30 minutes, 3 days per week during the 4-week course of radiotherapy. Control patients were advised to rest if they became fatigued. The aerobic exercise produced significant improvement in physical functioning, with no significant increase in fatigue in patients, while patients in the control group reported increased fatigue from baseline to completion of radiotherapy.

There is accumulating evidence on the importance of exercise in reducing cancer risk. Evidence is particularly strong for colon cancer, but data also suggest decreased risk of breast cancer in women who exercised, particularly during their late childhood and early adulthood. The effects of exercise on cancer may be related to reducing obesity. Current American Cancer Society guidelines suggest physical activity of at least moderate intensity for at 30 minutes on five of more days of the week.

Many additional studies of cancer patients and healthy individuals document the value of exercise. Tai chi, qigong, and yoga are especially suitable for cancer patients at various stages of disease.

TAI CHI

Tai chi is an ancient Chinese exercise program that incorporates movement, meditation, and breathing. Its motions reflect the yin–yang balance so fundamental to traditional Chinese medicine (see Chapter 2). Tai chi is well documented to improve muscle tone, agility, balance, and flexibility. The practice of breathing exercises may serve a meditative function, thereby promoting stress reduction. Tai chi is particularly suited for older people and patients, as its movements are gentle and it puts less stress on the body than do other exercises.

Studies document the benefits of tai chi, including producing significant reductions in falls and hip fractures in older people and lowered heart rate and blood pressure in patients after heart attack. A randomized trial of 132 postmenopausal women showed that tai chi retarded bone loss. Tai chi is very gentle and therefore suitable even for frail patients.

QIGONG

Qigong is a moderate exercise regimen that emphasizes controlled breathing. Clinically able cancer patients usually prefer it to the gentler tai chi. It too reduces stress and anxiety, induces a sense of well-being and improves overall physical fitness, balance, and flexibility. Recent reviews of qigong trials, most of which were conducted in China, suggest that qigong may lead to improvements in cancer patients' quality of life and well being, for example, by reducing pain of anxiety. Additional research is needed to confirm these findings. Meanwhile, qigong is associated with minimal risk and the potential of substantial benefit. Moreover, patients typically enjoy and welcome qigong and tai chi.

YOGA

Yoga, a 5,000-year-old exercise regimen developed in India, also involves proper breathing, movement, and posture. Research documents its value in improving physical fitness and decreasing respiratory rate and blood pressure; yoga is often part of integrative management for heart disease, asthma, diabetes, drug addition, acquired immunodeficiency syndrome (AIDS), migraine headaches, and arthritis, as well as cancer.

A randomized clinical trial of 39 lymphoma patients evaluated the effectiveness of Tibetan yoga, which incorporates controlled breathing, visualization, mindfulness, and low-impact postures. Patients under treatment or who had concluded treatment in the prior 12 months participated in seven weekly sessions. Researchers concluded that the yoga program significantly improved sleep-related outcomes, including better quality, longer duration, and decreased use of sleep medications. In another study, 59 breast cancer patients and 10 prostate cancer patients participated in an 8-week mindfulness-based stress reduction (MBSR) program (see Chapter 7) that incorporated yoga as well as relaxation and meditation. Patients were assessed before and after the intervention. Although no significant improvement in mood disturbance emerged, the MBSR program significantly enhanced patients' quality of life and decreased symptoms of stress.

MASSAGE THERAPIES

Massage involves various manipulative techniques that touch the skin in comforting ways and move muscles and soft tissues. Massage therapy uses varying degrees of pressure, depending on the patient's clinical status, to reduce tension and pain, improve circulation, and encourage relaxation. It has important emotional and psychological benefits and is used as a complementary adjunct in the treatment of many illnesses. Massage therapies are especially valued by cancer patients. They help treat lymphedema following lymph node dissection, muscle tension, insomnia, pain, anxiety and depression, and sleeplessness.

TYPES OF MASSAGE

- **Swedish massage**, the most common, is comprised of five basic strokes and their variations.
- **Shiatsu**, from Japan, involves deep pressure to specific acupoints and often is too strong for cancer patient management. **Deep tissue massage** similarly applies strong finger pressure to release chronic muscle tension.
- **Reiki** is a controversial technique involving the "transmission of healing energy" from practitioner to patient. It comes originally from the Japanese healing tradition and more recently from North American nursing.
- **Reflexology** (foot massage), a soothing intervention, is often preferred by patients who are frail or terminally ill.
- **Rolfing** involves application of deep pressure to loosen fascia, aims to restore proper body alignment. It involves more pressure than is safe for cancer patients.
- **Tuina,** a Chinese massage technique, stimulates specific acupuncture points and is said to reduce symptoms and promote healing.

A randomized crossover study of 230 cancer patients receiving chemotherapy evaluated the effects of massage therapy and healing touch. Patients received a total of four weekly 45-minute sessions of massage, healing touch, or personal visit without therapy. Results showed that both massage therapy and healing touch reduced blood pressure, respiratory rate, and heart rate. Pain, mood disturbance, and fatigue decreased. Patients receiving massage therapy used less nonsteroidal anti-inflammatory medication. In another randomized trial, 42 patients with advanced cancer were randomized to receive weekly massage for 4 weeks. Patients experienced significant improvement in sleep and significant reduction in the depression scores.

A crossover study of 23 inpatients with breast or lung cancer evaluated anxiety and pain following reflexology (foot massage). Patients experienced significant decreases in anxiety. On one of three pain measures, breast cancer patients experienced significant decreases in pain as well. Research also shows that massage therapy reduces anxiety in infants and children with various medical conditions.

READINGS AND RESOURCES

1. Carlson LE, Speca M, Patel KD, Goodey E. Minfulness-based stress reduction in relation to quality of life, mood, symptoms of stress and levels of cortisol, dehydroepiandrosterone sulfate (DHEAS) and melatonin in breast and prostate cancer patients. Psychoneuroendocrinology 2004;29:448–74.
2. Cassileth BR, Vickers AJ. Massage therapy for symptom control: outcome study at a major cancer center. J Pain Sympt Manage 2004;28:244–49.
3. Cohen L, Warneke C, Fouladi RT, et al. Psychological adjustment and sleep quality in a randomized trial of the effects of a Tibetan yoga intervention in patients with lymphoma. Cancer 2004;100:2253–60.
4. Marchese VG, Chiarello LA, Lange BJ. Effects of physical therpy intervention for children with acute lymphoblastic leukemia. Pediatr Blood Cancer 2004;42:127–33.

10

Using the Senses

Our five senses enable us to process information and to benefit from positive aspects of the outside world. Conscious attention to that information can help cancer patients by providing distraction from frightening, unwanted thoughts and by enabling thorough relaxation. Engaging one or more of the senses, these therapies allow a restful and fulfilling experience, and they offer patients who want it an active role in their own care.

These complementary therapies clearly do not cure or treat underlying disease. They are, however, noninvasive, pleasant ways to help live productively and more comfortably through the strains of cancer diagnosis and treatment, and they provide satisfying, meaningful clinical benefit. Anecdotally, simultaneous use of as many senses as possible, such as having a warm bath with fragrant bath oils while listening to soft music and imagining a place of calm and beauty, seems to magnify the benefit.

MUSIC THERAPY

Today, more than 5,000 professional music therapists work in health care settings in the United States. In Canada, music therapists work in special schools and prisons, as well as hospitals and cancer centers. Music appears to benefit patients of all ages and clinical circumstances. Music therapists play a special role as members of cancer management teams in many oncology programs.

Frequently available in cancer centers, music therapy is applied to reduce anxiety and depression and promote general well-being. It is also thought to alleviate pain. Several studies show that music therapy is an effective complementary technique in various settings. A randomized, controlled clinical trial of 69 patients awaiting autologous stem cell transplantation for hematologic malignancies found that music therapy significantly reduced mood disturbance.

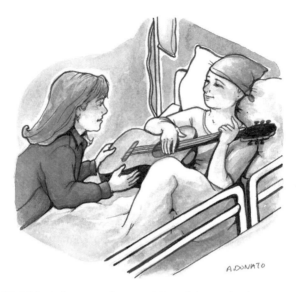

Figure 10-1 Music therapy reduces anxiety and depression in cancer patients.

Music therapy improved quality of life in a clinical trial of 80 end-stage cancer patients and reduced anxiety in patients receiving radiation therapy for pelvic or abdominal malignancies. Premature babies exposed to music in intensive care units were discharged more quickly, and music reduced anxiety in children undergoing surgical and medical procedures. Research also supports the ability of music therapy to reduce self-reported levels of dental and postoperative pain as well as the amount of anesthesia required during labor.

ART THERAPY

Based on the belief that the creative process is intrinsically therapeutic, art therapy applies creative activity as a rehabilitation technique for the sick and disabled. By allowing patients to express hidden emotions, it is believed to facilitate physical, mental, and spiritual healing. For patients who cannot themselves create, appreciating works of art by others can produce similar benefits. The visual images created by the patient provide a tangible, permanent record of the patient's state of mind at that time and allow the therapist, artist, nurse, or educator to access the patient's emotions.

Although proponents of art therapy claim that it promotes healing, there is little documentation of art therapy's benefits in the medical literature. Publications consist primarily of descriptive reports and suggest benefits for psychiatric patients and those suffering from chronic stress, serious illness, and Alzheimer's disease.

A clinical trial involving 32 pediatric leukemia patients, aged 2 to 14 years, found art therapy useful in preventing permanent trauma during painful procedures. Many medical centers and cancer programs hold art exhibitions, organize art workshops, or enable expressive art activities for patients. Such activities are believed to foster physical, mental, and spiritual healing and to contribute to the well-being of patients and caregivers.

AROMATHERAPY

Aromatherapy is the use of essential oils derived from distillation of plants for therapeutic purposes. The oils are applied on the skin as massage oils or inhaled directly from a saturated gauze pad placed beneath the patients' nostrils or through vaporizers or hot water baths. Aromatherapy is thought to aid stress reduction, prevent disease, and treat physical ailments such as acne, cold and flu, skin disorders, muscle tension, premenstrual disorders, and pain. It is also believed to help alleviate mental ailments such as anxiety, mild depression, dementia, and insomnia.

Studies using aromatherapy for palliative care in cancer patients show that it improves quality of life. But results from a placebo-controlled, double-blind, randomized trial involving 313 patients indicate that aromatherapy is not beneficial in reducing anxiety during radiotherapy. Other studies using massage in cancer patients found that the addition of essential oils enhances the therapeutic effects of massage. Evidence, however, is lacking in other minor and self-limiting conditions such as headaches and colds, which proponents claim can be treated by aromatherapy.

Ingredients in some of the essential oils may cause allergic reactions or trigger asthmatic attacks. Aromatherapy is contraindicated in patients who are sensitive to these ingredients. Although some oils are selected for their antiseptic properties, it is prudent not to use undiluted essential oils on open wounds. Essential oils are indicated only for topical use. Like other complementary methods, aromatherapy can affect a sense of relaxation and a calming atmosphere.

DANCE THERAPY

Dance therapy is the use of dance or rhythmic motion to assist healing and enhance well-being. Proponents believe that body and mind are inseparable and that body movement reflects inner emotional state. Physical motion provides the benefits of exercise and also appears to encourage positive thoughts and emotions that may contribute to growth and well-being. The medical literature contains articles on the benefits of dance therapy for adolescent and adult psychiatric patients, the elderly, and children and adults with mental or physical handicaps. Because dance or movement therapy helps overcome feelings of isolation and motivates social relationships in a group setting, it also encourages social interaction and creative expression, enhancing quality of life.

Many cancer programs include dance or movement therapies. An example, jointly run by the Singapore General Hospital and Singapore's Breast Cancer Foundation, is a dance therapy group established in the belief that dance therapy provides exercise, improves mobility, muscle coordination, body image, and self-esteem and reduces muscle tension, stress, anxiety, isolation, and chronic pain. Gentle exercise of this kind is beneficial in the pediatric and adult cancer setting.

HUMOR THERAPY

Humor or laughter therapy is the deliberate use of humor as a complementary treatment for people suffering from physical or emotional disorders. Humor can facilitate symptom relief by distracting the patient from constant awareness of pain. It is also believed to improve emotional and psychological health by encouraging stress reduction. Humor therapy is often made available to children and adult cancer patients as well as to those suffering from depression, the elderly in nursing homes, and cardiac patients.

Despite the absence of studies that document the healing powers of humor therapy, research has documented the physiologic effects of laughter. Laughing lowers blood pressure, increases muscle flexibility, and releases endorphins. It also may increase immune activity and reduce levels of cortisol, the stress hormone associated with immune suppression. According to a National Institutes of Health survey, 19% of comprehensive cancer centers, so designated by the National Cancer Institute, offer humor therapy.

READINGS AND RESOURCES

1. Cassileth BR, Vickers AJ, Magill LA. Music therapy for mood disturbance during hospitalization for autologous stem cell transplantation: a randomized controlled trial. Cancer 2003;98:2723–9.

Part II

COMPLEMENTARY THERAPIES BY CANCER DIAGNOSIS

Most complementary therapies are not specific to a particular cancer diagnosis. Instead, they are used typically to treat symptoms shared by patients across most cancer diagnoses. This is generally appropriate, as symptoms tend to stem less from the diagnosis than from toxicities associated with treatment or metastatic disease, which evoke similar symptoms in patients across cancer diagnoses. Chemotherapy-induced nausea and vomiting, for example, is associated more closely with the emetogenic potency of the drug used than with the underlying cancer diagnosis.

However, some symptoms are more prevalent in patients with particular cancers, owing either to the pathophysiology of the disease or to the treatment regimen. For example, intractable pain is more likely in patients with advanced pancreatic cancer, and postmenopausal symptoms occur more often in breast cancer patients on hormonal therapy. Evidence-based integrative therapies that reduce these and other symptoms are discussed in this section.

Breast cancer in women or prostate cancer in men along with lung cancer and colorectal cancer occupy the top three slots in terms of numbers of new cases and deaths, according to 2004 American Cancer Society estimates. The following four chapters address complementary therapies for prevention, treatment, and symptom control in these most common cancers.

11

Breast Cancer

PREVALENCE

Estimates for use of complementary and alternative medicine (CAM) among cancer patients in general range from 57% to over 80%; the variation is accounted for by researchers' varying definitions of CAM. Percentages are high among breast cancer patients. A survey in Vermont showed that 72% of breast cancer patients used at least one CAM treatment; vitamins and nonfood supplements were most common. A survey in San Francisco revealed variation by ethnicity, with blacks prone to spiritual healing, Chinese patients selecting herbal remedies, Latino women using dietary therapies and spiritual healing, and whites primarily using dietary methods and physical modalities such as massage therapy and acupuncture.

A Canadian survey of breast cancer survivors showed that 67% of respondents used CAM, most commonly in hopes of boosting immune function and to improve quality of life. In these and other studies, about one-half of patients indicate that they discussed CAM use with their physicians.

Breast cancer patients tend to be actively involved in their treatment, seeking and exploring information. Many learn about CAM through exchanges in support groups or others' efforts to "do everything possible to fight the cancer." In addition, large numbers of patients become breast cancer survivors thanks to early detection and advances in treatment. These women tend to be very health conscious and eager to explore the role of complementary therapies in long-term health maintenance.

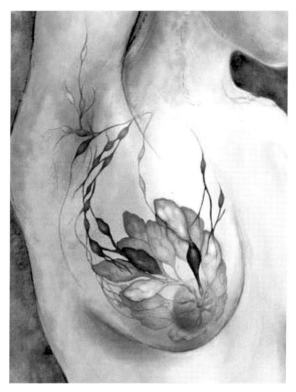

Figure 11-1 Lymphatic drainage of the breast: typical routes of tumor spread.

BREAST CANCER PREVENTION

Diet

Some dietary regimens, such as the Gerson and macrobiotic diets (see Chapters 5 and 19), are promoted as viable cancer treatment options, but neither they nor any other dietary approach is an effective treatment for cancer. Diet, however, can play an important role in cancer prevention.

In general, high saturated fat and high caloric intake are associated with higher cancer risk. Epidemiologic studies show that Asian-American women born in the West have a greater risk for breast cancer risk than do Asian-American women born in the East.

Although most animal studies show that dietary fat increases the development of breast tumors, data from case-control or cohort human studies are less strong. Type of fat is important, as studies show an inverse relationship between consumption of olive oil (monounsaturated fat) or fish oil (polyunsaturated fat) and breast cancer risk.

Epidemiologic as well as animal studies support the importance of fruits and vegetables, as they too decrease breast cancer risk. Excess body weight is a significant risk factor for recurrence and for shorter survival in breast cancer patients. This relationship is most substantial in stage 1 and 2 patients. Given other health benefits such as reduced risk of cardiovascular disease and diabetes, a high fruits and vegetables, low saturated fat diet is advisable. Several current clinical trials—the Women's Health Initiative (WHI), the Women's Intervention Nutrition Study (WINS), and the Women's Healthy Eating and Lifestyle Study (WHEL)—further address the relationship between dietary fat, other components of diet, and the risk of breast cancer and other diseases. Results are expected in 2006.

Dairy Products

Breast cancer patients often ask whether they should eliminate dairy products from their diets, as an old idea newly surfaced in the "alternative" medicine community suggests. A book based on one woman's experience following her mainstream breast cancer treatment indicates that dairy products are high in saturated fat, hormones, and pesticides, which increase breast cancer risk. Research evidence, unfortunately, is unclear. Some data suggest that calcium, vitamin D, and conjugated linoleic acid in dairy products can reduce the risk, while others show higher, lower, or absent breast cancer risk in relation to dairy foods.

A confounding issue in some reports on dairy products and breast cancer is researchers' failure to control for the fat content of dairy products consumed by study participants. The consumption of full-fat milk, cottage cheese, and other dairy products is likely to increase weight and, along with it, the breast cancer risk associated with obesity. Women who consume low- or no-fat products may retain the benefits of calcium and others components while avoiding excess fat consumption. It is reasonable for women not to avoid dairy products but to adopt low-fat products as part of a healthy lifestyle.

Soy Products

Breast cancer is less common in Asian countries, where more soy and soy products are consumed. Some research suggests that soy products may decrease breast cancer risk. Soy contains isoflavones such as genistein and daidzein that may interact with estrogen receptors. These phytoestrogen isoflavones produce both estrogenic and antiestrogenic effects in vitro. The effect may depend on the concentration or other cofactors in the cells, not unlike other selective estrogen receptor modulators (SERMs).

In animal studies, feeding rats soy-enriched diets through puberty reduced the incidence of mammary tumors later in life. Such an effect was not seen when the special diet was started after puberty. Epidemiologic studies in general fail to show a protective effect for soy products, except in women who consume them during adolescence or in large amounts. Based on existing data, the consumption of soy products in moderation is neither encouraged nor discouraged for the prevention of breast cancer. Following breast cancer diagnosis, however, additional factors come into play.

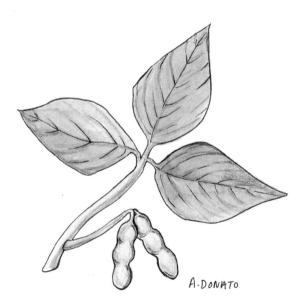

Figure 11-2 Abundant use of soy products should be avoided by women with ER+ breast cancer.

The phytoestrogen activity in soy products raises concerns about their use by breast cancer patients or survivors with estrogen receptor positive cancer. In theory, these products may increase the risk of breast cancer recurrence or progression. It is prudent for these women to refrain from concentrated soy products, such as soy powder, soy supplements, or more than three half-cup servings of tofu, soy milk, or other soy products per week.

DURING TREATMENT

It is prudent to advise patients not to use herbal products during treatment. Herbal products usually have poorly defined and inconsistent chemical constituents, making their biologic effects less than predictable. Some herbal products interact with anesthetics or anticoagulants, creating potential perioperative problems. Others modulate the expression and activity of cytochrome P-450 (CYP) enzymes, leading to altered pharmacokinetics of chemotherapeutic agents (see Chapter 4).

Herbs such as *Trifolium pratense* (red clover) and *Humulus lupulus* (hops) have moderate estrogenic activity, whereas *Angelica sinensis* (Dong Guai) and *Glycyrrhiza glabra* (licorice) show weak estrogen-receptor binding affinity. These products should be avoided in estrogen-receptor–positive breast cancer patients.

The use of antioxidant supplements during cancer treatment is controversial. Some data suggest that antioxidants reduce side effects without compromising treatment efficacy, while other studies show that they may interfere with radiation or chemotherapy. Until definitive data become available, it is prudent to avoid high-dose antioxidants during radiation therapy and certain classes of chemotherapy, such as alkylating agents (cyclophosphamide and platins) or anthracyclines (doxorubicin and epirubicin), given the uncertain and moderate, if any, benefits and the potential adverse effects on treatment efficacy. Other complementary therapies that can safely relieve side effects during breast cancer treatment are discussed below.

Chemotherapy-Induced Nausea and Vomiting

Some chemotherapeutic agents used in breast cancer treatment, such as cyclophosphamide, methotrexate, and doxorubicin, are highly emetogenic. Acupuncture can help relieve chemotherapy-induced nausea and vomiting. The PC 6 acupuncture point, located about two inches superior to the transverse crease of the wrist, between the tendons of muscles palmaris longus and flexor carpi radialis, is the most commonly used and best studied point for nausea and vomiting.

Electroacupuncture at PC 6 has been shown to reduce both nausea and the number of emetic episodes in breast cancer patients receiving myeloablative chemotherapy. In this randomized trial, electroacupuncture was superior to both a placebo acupuncture technique and to no acupuncture. All patients received the antiemetics prochlorperazine, lorazepam, and diphenhydramine. Acupuncture has also been shown to help relieve nausea and vomiting associated with pregnancy and surgery.

The combination of acupuncture with serotonin receptor antagonists, the newest generation of antiemetics, was tested recently. In a trial of patients with rheumatic disease, the combination decreased the severity of nausea and the number of vomiting episodes more than ondansetron alone in patients receiving methotrexate (an agent also used in chemotherapy). However, a study of cancer patients reported no improvement for ondansetron plus acupuncture versus ondansetron plus placebo acupuncture. Given the excellent antiemetic effect of the serotonin receptor antagonists, it is unlikely that acupuncture would produce major additional benefit. However, it is reasonable to offer acupuncture to patients with difficult-to-control chemotherapy-induced nausea and vomiting.

The mechanism of action of acupuncture is under investigation. Modulation of cerebellar activity was observed in a functional magnetic resonance imaging study of PC 6 acupuncture, suggesting that the effect may be mediated via the cerebellar vestibular neuromatrix.

Anthracycline Cardiotoxicity

Anthracyclines such as doxorubicin can cause early cardiomyopathy and late-onset ventricular dysfunction many years after the completion of treatment. The cardiotoxicity is often a dose-limiting adverse effect and can have major negative impact on quality of life. Dose reduction and change of drug formulation and delivery method may reduce the risk of this complication, but this also may risk decreased antineoplastic effect.

Because oxidative stress is one of the proposed mechanisms of anthracycline-induced cardiotoxicity, metal ion chelators and free radical scavengers have been studied as cardioprotectors. An iron chelator, dexrazoxane, appears to reduce free radical generation by anthracyclines. This agent was shown to protect against doxorubicin-induced cardiomyopathy. However, because of concerns about interference with the antitumor efficacy of anthracyclines, it is approved by the U.S. Food and Drug Administration (FDA) only for women with metastatic breast cancer who received a cumulative doxorubicin dose of 300 mg/m^2 and who would benefit from continuing therapy with doxorubicin. It is not recommended for use with initiation of doxorubicin therapy.

Based on a similar rationale, other antioxidants have been studied as cardioprotectors. Despite concerns about interactions, many antioxidants are advocated for the prevention and treatment of cardiomyopathy. Coenzyme Q10 (ubiquinone; known as Co-Q10) is perhaps the most advertised and the most commonly used by patients. Most studies of Co-Q10 were conducted to address congestive heart failure in general and not anthracycline-induced heart failure in particular. Although preclinical studies and several small clinical trials suggested its effectiveness, other clinical trials showed no effect. A recent randomized controlled study tested the effect of Co-Q10 at 200 mg per day in 55 patients with congestive heart failure. No significant difference in ejection fraction, peak oxygen consumption, and exercise duration were observed, indicating that co-enzyme Q10 is not an effective treatment for congestive heart failure. No clinical trial shows that ubiquinone prevents anthracycline-induced cardiomyopathy without compromising antineoplastic efficacy.

L-Carnitine is another free radical scavenger involved in mitochondrial function. It is approved by the FDA for primary or secondary carnitine deficiency but is also available as a dietary supplement. It was reported to improve the performance of patients with congestive heart failure in a few clinical studies, but a subsequent multicenter, randomized, placebo-controlled trial conducted in more than 500 patients with mild to moderate congestive heart failure patients treated with angiotensin-converting enzyme (ACE) inhibitors and diuretics found no significant difference in maximum exercise duration. Subanalysis showed statistically significant improvement in maximum exercise duration in patients with a higher (> 30%) ejection fraction. No safety issue was encountered. This agent may be of value in select patients. Further study in anthracycline-treated patients with mild or subclinical cardiomyopathy appears to be warranted.

Paclitaxel Neuropathy

Taxanes, especially paclitaxel, can cause polyneuropathy. The incidence and severity of neuropathy appear to be related to dose level and cumulative dose. It usually manifests as a predominant sensory distal neuropathy in fingers and toes. In some patients, this neuropathy becomes a dose-limiting toxicity and lasts beyond the treatment period.

L-Glutamine is one of few agents that showed promise as a prophylaxis for paclitaxel-induced neuropathy. Glutamine, a nonessential amino acid, is available as a dietary supplement. Animal studies suggest it protects the host during radiation and chemotherapy without increasing the resistance of tumor to treatment. A paired pre- and postpaclitaxel evaluation of patients receiving high-dose paclitaxel was conducted. Oral glutamine was given at 10 g three times daily for 4 days starting 24 hours after completion of high-dose paclitaxel. Significant reduction in the severity of peripheral neuropathy was observed. This phase II trial was limited by lack of placebo control and by extremely high doses of paclitaxel. The benefit of glutamine for patients receiving standard-dose paclitaxel is unknown. A prospective randomized evaluation of oral glutamine as a neuroprotectant in patients receiving weekly standard doses of paclitaxel is underway.

Trastuzumab (Herceptin) and glucans

Trastuzumab is a humanized monoclonal antibody specific to the human epidermal growth factor receptor 2 (HER2) protein. It is approved for the treatment of metastatic breast cancer in select patients. There are investigational efforts to enhance its efficacy by coadministering β-glucan. β-Glucans are present in many polysaccharide extracts from barley, yeast, and mushrooms. The extracts, available as dietary supplements, are advocated to boost immune function. Animal studies show that oral administration of β-glucan can synergize the antitumor effect of monoclonal antibodies, probably through enhancement of antibody-dependent cell-mediated cyto-toxicity. A few clinical studies combining monoclonal antibody with glucans are underway. It will be interesting to see what effects and adverse effects will result from this combination and whether it has a viable role in the treatment of breast cancer.

Radiation Dermatitis

Some cancer patients use topical botanical products, such as aloe vera or calendula, to reduce dermatitis caused by radiation thera-py. A clinical study showed that aloe vera gel was not better than placebo or aqueous cream in reducing radiation-induced dermatitis. Aloe vera gel added to soap has a stronger protective effect than soap alone in patients receiving high cumulative radiation doses. Calendula, derived from the marigold flower, is often used for wound healing. It may have anti-inflammatory activity. A recent phase III randomized trial in France found that calendula prevents acute der-matitis related to radiation therapy in breast cancer patients. Both aloe vera and calendula can cause allergic reactions in some patients.

AFTER TREATMENT

Osteoporosis

Breast cancer survivors are at a high risk of osteoporosis. In double-blind, randomized controlled trials, soy isoflavones helped maintain bone-mineral density among women without cancer, including older postmenopausal women, those with lower body weight, and women with lower levels of calcium intake in one study but not in another, both published in 2004. One randomized crossover trial in post-menopausal women with a history of breast cancer found that bone resorption markers were reduced significantly in women using phy-toestrogens (isoflavonoids) versus placebo. Bone formation markers were not affected. However, estrogen replacement therapy is com-monly contraindicated in these women. The concern that phytoe-strogens stimulate the growth of breast cancer cells renders the use of phytoestrogens problematic.

Increased intake of foods rich in calcium and vitamin D, as well as calcium and vitamin D supplementation, helps prevent osteo-porosis. Exercise, especially weight-bearing exercise, is also helpful. Tai chi chuan, a form of martial arts emphasizing slow, gentle, and fluid movements, was tested in a randomized prospective trial that found significantly less bone density loss compared with sedentary-lifestyle women. Because tai chi chuan provides other benefits such as improved physical function, sleep quality, and fall fracture prevention, this type of exercise regimen can be particularly beneficial to older women.

Hot Flashes

Women with natural or oophorectomy-, chemotherapy-, or tamoxifen-induced menopause can develop vasomotor symptoms such as hot flashes. Symptoms may be severe enough to interfere with sleep or daily functioning. Acupuncture, mind–body techniques, and vitamin E supplementation have been studied for postmenopausal symptoms. Phytoestrogen extracts from soy or red clover were investigated in two large randomized, controlled trials. Neither showed clinically meaningful efficacy against hot flashes (see Chapter 18).

Lymphedema

Lymphedema affected by axillary lymph node dissection causes discomfort and disability of the arm, increased risk of infection, and body image concerns. Compression bandaging, sequential pneumatic compression, or containment garment are used to reduce the arm swelling. Manual therapy has been tested alone and in combination with other interventions.

Manual lymphatic drainage (MLD), which provides gentle pumping action through specific hand movements, helps breast cancer-related lymphedema. In a randomized controlled crossover study, the effects of MLD were compared with those of simple lymphatic drainage, a less robust massage regimen, in 31 women with breast cancer-related lymphedema. MLD significantly reduced excess limb volume and dermal thickness and significantly improved quality-of-life endpoints.

MLD was compared in a randomized study with sequential pneumatic compression (SPC) as maintenance therapy after an initial 2 weeks of therapy with a standard compression sleeve. Both MLD and SPC reduced lymphedema, but only the MLD group reported a further decrease of tension and heaviness. MLD combined with multilayered compression bandaging (CB) was compared with CB alone in another randomized trial. CB, with or without MLD, was effective in reducing arm lymphedema volume. Combined MLD and CB works best in women with mild lymphedema.

Supplementation of selenium, a functional component of antioxidant enzymes, may help relieve lymphedema. In a randomized, placebo-controlled, double-blind study with postmastectomy lymphedema patients undergoing combined physical decongestion therapy (CPDT), sodium selenite increased the efficacy of CPDT, reduced edema volume, and improved mobility and heat tolerance in the affected extremity. Selenium also reduced radiation-associated lymphedema in limbs as well as in the head and neck region.

Proposed mechanisms include maintaining membrane integrity via redox modulation, suppressing adhesion and clogging of lymphocytes to lymphatic microcapillaries, and enhancing degradation of excess tissue proteins by macrophages. The good safety profile of selenium and its cost effectiveness make it an attractive addition to the management of lymphedema.

READINGS AND RESOURCES

1. Kaptchuk TJ. Acupuncture: theory, efficacy, and practice. Ann Intern Med 2002;136:374–83.
2. Kronenberg F, Fugh-Berman A. Complementary and alternative medicine for menopausal symptoms: a review of randomized, controlled trials. Ann Intern Med 2002;137:805–13.
3. Ladas EJ, Jacobson JS, Kennedy DD, Teel K, Fleischauer A, Kelly KM. Antioxidants and cancer therapy: a systematic review. *J Clin Oncol.* Feb 1 2004;22(3):517-528.
4. Sparreboom A, Cox MC, Acharya MR, Figg WD. Herbal remedies in the United States: potential adverse interactions with anticancer agents. J Clin Oncol 2004;22:2489–503.
5. Tretli S, Haldorsen T, Ottestad L. The effect of pre-morbid height and weight on the survival of breast cancer patients. Br J Cancer 1990;62:299–303.

12

Gastrointestinal Cancers

Colorectal cancer is the third most commonly diagnosed and the third most deadly cancer in the United States. More people die of digestive system cancers, which include liver and pancreatic cancers, than any other except for lung cancer. About one-half of colorectal cancer patients use complementary therapies according to a Canadian study; close to 70% informed their physicians. There has been extensive research on complementary therapies in the prevention of gastrointestinal (GI) cancers and their role in reducing side effects during and after treatment.

PREVENTION

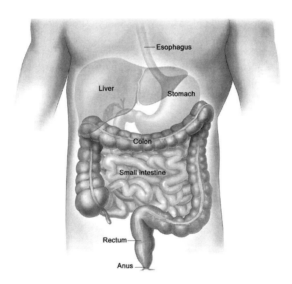

Figure 12-1 Complementary therapies are under study for the prevention of GI cancers.

Diet

Diet plays an important role in the prevention of GI cancers. Convincing evidence indicates that obesity increases the risk of esophageal and colon cancers, high alcohol intake elevates the risk of esophageal and liver cancers, and ingestion of aflatoxin-contaminated peanuts or grains increases the risk of liver cancer. Salt-preserved foods and high salt intake are linked to stomach cancer. However, dietary fiber significantly lowers the risk of colon cancer. Therefore, a low-fat diet high in fruits, vegetables, and fiber diet is advisable, especially considering the many other benefits of such a diet (see Chapter 5).

Dietary Supplements

Most supplement research addresses chemopreventive agents, with primary emphasis on colorectal cancer and precancerous adenoma. Calcium may lower the risk of colorectal adenomas by suppressing cell proliferation. Increasing the daily intake of calcium via low-fat dairy food reduces the proliferative activity of colonic epithelial cells and restores markers of normal cell differentiation in patients with a history of polypectomy for colonic adenomatous polyps. Recurrence of adenoma and the average number of adenomas were both significantly reduced by calcium intake in a large placebo-controlled, double-blind trial. In another large randomized intervention trial, calcium supplementation was associated with a modest but not significant reduction in risk of adenoma recurrence.

Folate intake is inversely associated with the risk of colorectal adenoma and cancer, as observed in both the Physicians' Health Study and the Nurses' Health Study. Although the chemopreventive effect has not been evaluated in placebo-controlled trials, folate supplementation should be considered given its low risk and the fact that many people do not have adequate folate intake through their regular diets.

Anti-inflammatory drugs such as nonsteroidal agents or cyclo-ogygenase-2 (COX-2) inhibitors also show promise in colon cancer prevention, and good evidence indicates that sulindac, aspirin, and celecoxib help prevent colonic adenomas. Some botanical products, such as turmeric, show anti-inflammatory activity as well as antitumor and antiangiogenesis activity in preclinical studies. Clinical trials evaluating the chemopreventive effect of curcumin, believed to be the active constituent in turmeric, are underway.

TJ-9

Liver cirrhosis progresses to hepatocellular carcinoma over time. TJ-9 (*Sho-saiko-to* in Japanese or *Xiao-chai-hu-tang* in Chinese) is an herbal formulation based on a traditional Chinese medicine recipe. It was evaluated as a chemopreventive agent in cirrhotic patients, where randomized controlled trials demonstrated that TJ-9 reduced the incidence of hepatocellular carcinoma and increased survival. This difference achieved statistical significance in hepatitis B surface (HBs) antigen–negative patients. The cancer-preventive effects are probably mediated by its antifibrotic activity. Clinical trials are under-way to investigate the ability of TJ-9 to suppress hepatitis C–induced cirrhosis.

DURING TREATMENT

5-Fluorouracil-Induced Mucositis

5-Fluorouracil (5-FU)-based regimens remain the most common adju-vant and palliative chemotherapy treatments for esophageal, gastric, and colorectal cancers. 5-FU can cause severe mucositis or stomati-tis, resulting in pain and malnourishment. Oral cooling is modestly helpful. Preemptive systemic or local administration of granulo-cyte/macrophage colony-stimulating factor (GM-CSF) can benefit some patients.

Glutamine, available as a dietary supplement, was studied for pos-sible ability to reduce chemotherapy-induced mucositis. Parental glu-tamine administration was not effective, but the application of oral topical glutamine significantly reduced the severity and duration of oral pain, as well as the length of restricted oral intake. Unfortunately, this benefit occurs only with some chemotherapy regimens, such as doxorubicin, etoposide, methotrexate, and ifosfamide. Two trials evaluating its effect with 5-FU-induced mucositis did not show a ben-efit.

A mouthwash containing chamomile extract was also tested with 5-FU regimens and found ineffective. Candy containing capsaicin, an extract of chili peppers, can produce temporary pain relief from chemotherapy-induced mucositis; investigators did not report the chemotherapy regimens studied. Tested in the stem cell transplantation setting, hypnotherapy (see Chapter 7) decreased mucositis pain more effectively than did standard care. Its utility against 5-FU-induced mucositis is unknown.

Irinotecan and Drug–Herb Interaction

Irinotecan, another agent commonly used to treat GI cancers, is metabolized by the cytochrome P-450 (CYP) 3A4 enzyme. The expression and function of this enzyme isoform is modulated by many agents, including botanical products. St. John's wort for depression, for example, is problematic when taken with some chemotherapeutic agents, as this herb induces the expression of CYP 3A4, resulting in reduced plasma levels of the active metabolite of irinotecan. Less myelosuppression occurred with irinotecan when St. John's wort was taken concurrently, but the plasma level of the active metabolite of irinotecan was also reduced, raising concerns about decreased antitumor effect. This illustrates the danger of concurrent use of chemotherapy and herbal products to reduce side effects, as herbal agents may actually lower chemotherapy's antitumor efficacy

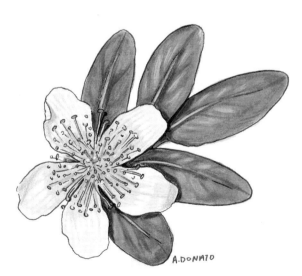

Figure 12-2 St. John's Wort induces CYP3A4 enzyme and can affect the metabolism of some pharmaceutical agents.

(see Chapter 4). Grapefruit juice is another dietary product that modulates CYP 3A4. It appears to inhibit the enteric 3A4 but not the hepatic component of drug metabolism, therefore having more effect on oral medications.

Coriolus versicolor

Also known as "turkey tail" or "Yun zhi," this mushroom is an important component of traditional Asian herbal remedies. Its extracts are used by some patients to boost immune function. The extracts polysaccharide K (PSK) and polysaccharide P (PSP) are polysaccharide peptide conjugates, primarily β-glucans, that are applied in Asia with chemotherapy to treat cancer. They display immunomodulatory activity in vitro and in animal studies. Controlled clinical trials conducted in Japan and China show benefits in cancer patients, especially those with GI cancers.

More than 200 stage 2 or 3 colorectal cancer patients were randomized to receive a fluorouracil-based oral agent with or without PSK as adjuvant therapy. Cancer recurrence, lung metastases, and disease-free and overall survivals were significantly better in the PSK

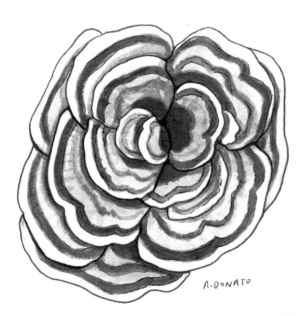

Figure 12-3 Extracts of Coriolus Versicolor may benefit patients with GI cancers.

group. The addition of PSK to chemotherapy after curative gastrectomy significantly improved 5-year disease-free survival and overall survival in gastric cancer patients. PSK also improved survival in esophageal cancer patients, although the improvement was not statistically significant. No benefit was found in hepatocellular carcinoma patients..

Coriolus extracts containing PSK and PSP are available in the United States as dietary supplements. It is uncertain how similar these products are to agents tested in the above clinical trials in terms of chemical composition and biological activity.

Virulizin

An extract of bovine bile, virulizin inhibits the growth of human pancreatic cancer cell xenograft in nude mice. It potentiates the effect of gemcitabine. In a phase II trial of 22 pancreatic cancer patients, virulizin did not cause tumor regression, but disease stabilization was observed for more than 3 months in six patients and for more than 15 months in two patients. Virulizin's effect is believed mediated by macrophage activity. A phase III randomized trial comparing gemcitabine plus virulizin with gemcitabine plus placebo is underway.

AFTER TREATMENT

Postoperative Recovery

Complementary therapies may aid recovery from abdominal surgery. Acupuncture, massage, and music therapies reduce postoperative pain (see Chapter 15), as well as nausea and vomiting (see Chapter 17).

Wound Healing

Hypnotherapy is used for pain reduction and procedural preparation. It was also studied for wound healing. A randomized trial compared the relative efficacy of an adjunctive hypnotic intervention against supportive attention and usual care in healthy women undergoing mammoplasty. Assessment by staff blinded to group assignment suggested accelerated wound healing in the hypnosis group. Although the sample was small, this provocative finding suggests that further study is worthwhile.

Dumping Syndrome

Esophagectomy or gastrectomy can produce dumping syndrome, with rapid transition of gastric content to the intestines and resulting abdominal cramps, diarrhea, and vasomotor symptoms such as diaphoresis, flushing, and dizziness. Dietary modification is important in managing this problem. Small, frequent meal of low carbohydrate content and the separation of liquid and solid intake are helpful. Because postprandial hyperglycemia promotes gastric motility, foods with low glycemic load and low glycemic index are advisable. Dietary supplements containing fiber, such as pectin, guar gum, and glucomannan, delay glucose absorption and prolong bowel transit time. On the other hand, diary products may exacerbate dumping syndrome.

Peppermint oil and caraway oil herbal supplements are sold as treatments for abdominal discomfort. Although neither delays gastric emptying, peppermint oil slowed intestinal transit in a study of healthy volunteers. Omega-3 fatty acids, found in fish oil, flaxseed oil, and borage oil supplements, can cause rapid gastric emptying and should be avoided by these patients.

An herbal preparation containing yerba maté (leaves of *Ilex paraguayensis*), seeds of guarana (*Paullinia cupana*), and leaves of damiana (*Turnera diffusa* and *T. aphrodisiaca*) was tested in a trial of healthy volunteers and found to delay gastric emptying more effectively than did placebo. Ginger root, although helpful for postoperative nausea and vomiting, does not appear to slow gastric emptying. Whether the results of these studies in healthy volunteers can be readily translated to patients with dumping syndrome has not been tested. There are no reports using acupuncture or mind–body techniques in treating dumping syndrome.

Dumping syndrome is alleviated by the following:
- Small, frequent meals
- Foods with low glycemic load and low glycemic index
- Fiber supplementation
- Separation of liquid and solid intake

Bowel Incontinence

Patients after colorectal or pelvic surgery may develop this problem. In addition to medical and surgical management, mind–body therapy can be helpful. Biofeedback in the treatment of fecal incontinence has been studied extensively. A 2001 meta-analysis of 35 studies found that most reported positive results for biofeedback, but additional quality research is lacking. More recent trials show inconsistent results regarding the efficacy of biofeedback when compared with other pelvic floor training techniques.

Pancreatic Cancer Cachexia

Patients with advanced cancer, especially pancreatic cancer, are prone to cachexia. Eicosapentaenoic acid (EPA), an omega-3 fatty acid found in fish oil supplements, stabilized the weight of pancreatic cancer patients who had lost weight in earlier studies. In an uncontrolled study of patients with other cancers who had lost weight in the proceeding month, weight stabilization was observed only in a minority of patients. These findings led to two large phase III studies. One showed that EPA alone or EPA plus megestrol acetate (Megace) was not superior to megestrol acetate alone in improving weight or appetite. Toxicities were similar except that more men reported impotence in the megestrol acetate groups. Whether pancreatic cancer patients were included in this trial is not clear.

Pancreatic Cancer Pain

Advanced pancreatic cancer can cause refractory pain via involvement of celiac plexus. Opioids or celiac block do not always provide satisfactory pain relief and are not always well tolerated. Acupuncture is under study for its potential to reduce this type of pain, as it may effectively treat neuropathic cancer pain. Results are pending.

READINGS AND RESOURCES

1. Heymen S, Jones KR, Ringel Y, et al. Biofeedback treatment of fecal incontinence: a critical review. Dis Colon Rectum 2001;44:728–36.
2. Jatoi A, Rowland K, Loprinzi CL, et al. An eicosapentaenoic acid supplement versus megestrol acetate versus both for patients with cancer-associated wasting: a North Central Cancer Treatment Group and National Cancer Institute of Canada collaborative effort. J Clin Oncol 2004;22:2469–76.

3. Mathijssen RH, Verweij J, de Bruijn P, et al. Effects of St. John's wort on irinotecan metabolism. J Natl Cancer Inst 2002;94:1247–9.
4. Ohwada S, Ikeya T, Yokomori T, et al. Adjuvant immunochemotherapy with oral Tegafur/Uracil plus PSK in patients with stage II or III colorectal cancer: a randomised controlled study. Br J Cancer 2004;90:1003–10.

13

Lung Cancer

No report focuses on the prevalence of complementary and alternative medicine (CAM) use in the lung cancer patient population specifically. Given the poor prognosis of advanced lung cancer despite current standards of care, it would not be surprising that many such patients explore CAM either as a last-resort treatment option or as an adjunct to improve quality of life. In addition, some people use CAM for health maintenance and cancer prevention. Because of promising data in preclinical studies, quite a few agents in the dietary supplement category have been studied in clinical trials for chemoprevention of lung cancer.

PREVENTION

Smoking Cessation

Smoking cessation has the largest impact in preventing lung cancer. Educational, behavioral, and medical interventions are the mainstay for smoking cessation. Some complementary modalities also have been applied to this effort.

Hypnosis is used to suppress the desire to smoke or to strengthen the will to stop. While some uncontrolled studies showed promising results, others produced conflicting results. When a rigorous criterion, such as abstinence at 6 months postintervention, was applied to a meta-analysis of nine randomized controlled trials, hypnotherapy did not demonstrate an effect superior to other interventions or to no treatment. Although hypnotherapy does not appear to improve quit rates, many studies report its ability to reduce cigarette consumption.

The effect of acupuncture has been studied, also with mixed results. A meta-analysis of 22 studies concluded that acupuncture was as effective as the many other interventions used for smoking cessation. A more recent randomized trial of 141 subjects tested auricular acupuncture, education, and the combination in achieving smoking cessation. The authors found that both modalities, alone or in combination, significantly reduced smoking. The combination showed a significantly greater effect in subjects with a greater pack-year history.

Brain imaging studies show that smoking suppresses blood flow to the anterior cingulate cortex, hippocampus, and amygdala. Curiously, these are the same areas suppressed by acupuncture. Given the huge public health impact of smoking and the imperfect results of existing smoking cessation techniques, further studies using refined acupuncture techniques guided by recent advances in acupuncture research are warranted.

> **Fruits and vegetables provide benefits that cannot be replaced by individual vitamin supplements.**

Diet and Dietary Supplements

The largest chemoprevention study to date is the Alpha-Tocopherol, Beta-Carotene (ATBC) Cancer Prevention Trial, a randomized controlled trial of 29,000 male smokers in Finland. Dietary supplementation with alpha-tocopherol, a form of vitamin E, or beta-carotene, a precursor of vitamin A, did not reduce the incidence of lung cancer among male smokers. On the contrary, beta-carotene was associated with increased risk of lung cancer, especially in current smokers and recent quitters. Both the beneficial and the adverse effects of supplemental alpha-tocopherol and beta-carotene disappeared during postintervention follow-up.

Further analysis of the dataset revealed additional findings. Although supplementation of alpha-tocopherol did not reduce overall incidence of lung cancer, higher serum alpha-tocopherol status was associated with lower lung cancer risk, particularly among younger persons and among those with less cumulative smoke exposure. This suggests that high levels of alpha-tocopherol, if present during the early critical stages of tumorigenesis, may inhibit lung cancer development.

An inverse association was identified between intake of flavonols (quercetin, myricetin, and kaempferol) and flavones (luteolin and apigenin) and the risk of lung, but not other, cancers. Onions, tea, and apples contained the highest amounts of flavonols and flavones. Analysis also showed that high fruit and vegetable consumption, particularly a diet rich in carotenoids, tomatoes, and tomato-based products, may reduce the risk of lung cancer.

In the Beta-Carotene and Retinol Efficacy Trial (CARET), another large chemoprevention trial of 18,000 smokers, former smokers, and workers exposed to asbestos, beta-carotene and vitamin A supplementation again was associated with a higher risk of lung cancer. Interestingly, subanalyses revealed that intake of fruits and vegetables was associated with reduced lung cancer risk only in the placebo arm. The association was strongest with rosaceae fruit or cruciferae vegetables. This illustrates that plant foods have an important role in preventing lung cancer in high-risk populations and that beta-carotene supplements do not provide the protective compounds found in plant foods.

Several agents have been tested for reversal of precancerous squamous metaplasia or dysplasia. Retinoids are ineffective. Vitamin B_{12} and folic acid showed some effects, albeit in a flawed study.

DURING TREATMENT

Pneumonitis and Fibrosis from Radiotherapy

Radiation therapy can cause pneumonitis and pulmonary fibrosis, especially when used with radiosensitizing agents. The administration of antioxidants to prevent such damage has been explored, the rationale being that antioxidants counteract the effect of reactive oxygen species generated by radiation. Because many dietary supplements have antioxidant properties, they are promoted by some people for reducing side effects of radiation therapy. Results from antioxidants found in food sources have not been strong. Antioxidant dietary supplements may have a stronger protective effect. Unfortunately the research is limited to a few reports of animal studies.

In a small single-arm study, supplementation with vitamins, trace elements, and fatty acids in combination with chemotherapy and irradiation appeared to prolong survival time in patients with small cell lung cancer. However, the control used was data from "most published combination treatment regimens alone," which is not a rigorous comparison. The concern has been that, if an antioxidant does not selectively protect normal cells better than it protects malignant cells, the antioxidant may reduce the efficacy of radiation treatment. A more promising approach, currently under study, is the use of agents such as amifostine, which show differential effects on normal versus malignant cells.

Platinum-Induced Neuropathy

Platinum-based agents, such as cisplatin and carboplatin, are first-line chemotherapies for the treatment of non–small cell lung cancer (NSCLC). They can cause dose-limiting peripheral neuropathy, and there is currently no evidence-based recommendation for the prophylaxis and treatment of oxaliplatin-induced neurotoxicity.

Several dietary supplements, including gingko extract, alpha-lipoic acid, and glutathione, have been studied for their potential to prevent platinum-induced neuropathy. Animal studies showed that gingko extract effectively reduces cisplatin-induced nerve damage, and a retrospective and a retrospective analyses found decreased duration and severity of oxaliplatin-induced neuropathy with the use of gingko extract.

In an uncontrolled study, alpha-lipoic acid was given to 14 patients who developed neuropathy on combined docetaxel and cisplatin. More than one-half of the patients reported improvement in neurologic symptoms. A randomized placebo-controlled trial showed that glutathione significantly reduced the incidence and severity of oxaliplatin-induced peripheral neuropathy in colorectal cancer patients. Deterioration of sural sensory nerve conduction was prevented by glutathione. The clinical activity of oxaliplatin was not reduced.

Cisplatin is highly ototoxic, causing hearing loss. N-acetyl-cysteine, another dietary supplement, was studied in vitro and in animal models and shown to protect against cisplatin-induced auditory neuronal and hair cell toxicity. Vitamin E, methionine, and glutathione ester also protect from cisplatin ototoxicity in animal models. No human study has been reported.

Sensory abnormalities caused by chemotherapy-induced neuropathy are different from neuropathic pain caused by direct nerve compression or inflitration by tumor. Athough acupuncture reduced neuropathic pain in cancer patients in a randomized controlled study, it is unclear how many of those patients had pain due to chemotherapy-induced neuropathy versus direct cancer involvement. However, acupuncture has been studied as a treatment for neuropathy in patients with human immunodeficiency virus (HIV) and diabetes. In a large, randomized study reported in 1998, neither acupuncture nor amitriptyline, a drug commonly prescribed for neuropathy, was more effective than placebo in relieving pain caused by HIV peripheral neuropathy. Because chemotherapy-induced neuropathy is caused by a different mechanism, additional research is required to determine whether acupuncture can reduce platinum- or taxane-related neuropathy.

Quality of life

Because the treatment of advanced lung cancer is largely palliative, adjunctive therapies to improve the quality of life of these patients would be clinically meaningful. Many complementary therapy regimens have been tested for this indication.

Mistletoe extract is popular in Europe. Although it may improve quality of life, it does not appear to exert a direct antitumor effect or to improve tumor response or survival. A 2003 systematic review of 23 mistletoe studies identified 12 with at least one statistically significant, positive result; 7 with at least one positive trend; 3 with no effect; and one with a negative trend. However, all studies suffered from methodologic shortcomings to some degree. Since then, a large, randomized controlled trial conducted under the auspices of the European Organization for Research and Treatment of Cancer (EORTC) found no benefit of mistletoe for the treatment of melanoma. Survival was slightly worse in patients receiving mistletoe compared to no treatment, and the investigators ruled out any clinical relevant benefit.

Hydrazine sulfate is another agent promoted by some as an alternative cancer therapy. An earlier randomized placebo-controlled study showed favorable although nonsignificant nutritional status and survival improvement in patients receiving hydrazine sulfate with platinum-based chemotherapy. These findings were not confirmed in subsequent studies. A phase III trial compared hydrazine sulfate versus placebo as an adjunct to cisplatin and vinblastine in the treatment of NSCLC. No significant difference in tumor survival, tumor response, nutritional status, or neuropathy emerged. Quality of life was significantly worse in the hydrazine sulfate group. Similarly, a study of newly diagnosed, unresectable NSCLC patients failed to show significant differences in survival, response, toxicity, or quality of life. Trends for worse time to progression and survival in the hydrazine sulfate arm were observed.

Dyspnea

Shortness of breath, or dyspnea, is a common symptom in cancer patients, particularly those with advanced cancer, where 50 to 70% experience significant symptoms. Patients with advanced lung cancer frequently develop dyspnea from parenchymal and pleural involvement of the cancer. High rates also occur in patients with other malignancies that metastasize to the lung. When the cancer is no longer responsive to treatment, relief from the sensation of air hunger becomes an important part of palliative care in these patients. Opioids are the primary treatment applied for this problem.

Because acupuncture has been shown to induce the production of endogenous opioids, it has been studied as a means of reducing dyspnea in lung cancer patients. An uncontrolled pilot study showed significant improvement in breathlessness scores, respiratory rate, relaxation, and anxiety. A systemic review suggests that patients with severe chronic obstructive pulmonary disease (COPD) may benefit from the use of acupuncture, acupressure, and muscle relaxation with breathing retraining to relieve dyspnea. However, data from two more recent controlled studies are less encouraging. Acupuncture was compared with a mock transcutaneous electrical nerve stimulation (TENS) unit as the placebo control in a crossover study for disabling, nonmalignant breathlessness, primarily COPD patients. Although breathlessness was significantly improved, no significant difference between the two interventions was found. A recent trial at Memorial Sloan-Kettering Cancer Center failed to find acupuncture superior to placebo for shortness of breath in patients with advanced cancer. Breathlessness scores fell immediately following acupuncture by about 20% in both groups, suggesting a placebo effect.

The subjective sensation of breathlessness correlates only poorly with oxygen saturation or pulmonary function. This suggests that shortness of breath has a cognitive component that might be addressed by behavioral intervention. Several randomized trials suggest that therapies involving a relaxation component, such as yoga or hypnosis, may relieve shortness of breath associated with asthma and COPD.

Accordingly, standard educational and rehabilitation programs for these disorders commonly incorporate advice about relaxation techniques. Such programs have also been developed for patients with cancer. A typical program includes assessment of factors that ameliorate or exacerbate shortness of breath, development of coping strategies, recognition of warning signs indicating the need for medical intervention, and training in breathing control techniques and relaxation. Such programs are of proven effectiveness in randomized trials. Relaxation techniques do not appear to have been evaluated as stand-alone interventions for shortness of breath in cancer patients.

AFTER TREATMENT

Postthoracotomy Pain

Thoracotomy commonly produces long-term pain at the operative site owing to injury to intercostal nerves. It is generally not severe but can be disabling in a small proportion of patients. Nonsteroidal anti-inflammatory medication, tricyclic antidepressants, and opioids are used as medical treatment, and nerve block is helpful in severe cases.

Nerve stimulation techniques such as TENS have been tested. In a phase III trial, TENS was found ineffective in the posterolateral thoracotomy group, which typically experiences severe pain. However, it was useful as an adjunct to medication in the muscle-sparing thoracotomy, costotomy, and sternotomy groups. For patients having video-assisted thoracoscopy, it was very effective as the only pain control treatment with no adjunct drugs.

Because acupuncture, another nerve stimulation technique, has been shown to relieve many pain conditions, it is under study as a treatment of thoracotomy pain in cancer patients. In this ongoing study, acupuncture treatment is delivered by small 2 mm needles affixed to perivertebral points preoperatively. The needles are left in place for another few weeks to provide continuous stimulation.

Prevention of Second Primary Tumor

Some lung cancer patients are at a higher risk of developing second primary tumors because of risk factors such as smoking. Several agents, mostly vitamin A class differentiating agents, have been tested for their preventative effect. High-dose vitamin A (retinyl palmitate) reduced the rate of second primary tumors following resection of early-stage primary lung cancer in a placebo-controlled trial. However, this finding was not confirmed in later trials, including the European Study on Chemoprevention with vitamin A and N-acetylcysteine (EUROSCAN), a large 2 × 2 trial. No significant differences in survival, event-free survival, or second primary tumors were observed.

Another retinoid, isotretinoin, was studied in a phase III trial. It failed to prevent second primary tumors in patients after complete resection of stage 1 NSCLC. Secondary analyses showed that isotretinoin was harmful in current smokers and beneficial in never smokers. Proposed explanations of this phenomenon include accelerated transformation by retinoic acid of cells with their genome already damaged by tobacco carcinogens and interaction of substances in tobacco smoke with retinoic acid resulting in a more powerful carcinogenic effect.

READINGS AND RESOURCES

1. The Alpha-Tocopherol, Beta Carotene Cancer Prevention Study Group. The effect of vitamin E and beta carotene on the incidence of lung cancer and other cancers in male smokers. N Engl J Med 1994;330:1029–35.
2. Cascinu S, Catalano V, Cordella L, et al. Neuroprotective effect of reduced glutathione on oxaliplatin-based chemotherapy in advanced colorectal cancer: a randomized, double-blind, placebo-controlled trial. J Clin Oncol 2002;20:3478–83.
3. Stauder H, Kreuser ED. Mistletoe extracts standardised in terms of mistletoe lectins (ML I) in oncology: current state of clinical research. Onkologie 2002;25:374–80.
4. van Zandwijk N, Dalesio O, Pastorino U, et al. EUROSCAN, a randomized trial of vitamin A and N-acetylcysteine in patients with head and neck cancer or lung cancer. For the European Organization for Research and Treatment of Cancer Head and Neck and Lung Cancer Cooperative Groups. J Natl Cancer Inst 2000;92:977–86.
5. White AR, Rampes H, Ernst E. Acupuncture for smoking cessation. Cochrane Database Syst Rev 2002;(2):CD000009.

14

Prostate Cancer

A growing number of patients with prostate cancer use complementary therapies, primarily herbal medicines. They are likely drawn in part because of substantial publicity about saw palmetto for benign prostate hypertrophy, PC SPES for prostate cancer, and the cancer prevention trials with selenium, vitamin E, and beta-carotene. Several surveys assessed prevalence of use by patients with prostate cancer and produced varied results depending on the definition of complementary and alternative medicine (CAM) applied by investigators. When spiritual practices such as prayer were included, 43% of those surveyed were found to use these modalities.

Patients use CAM remedies to suppress cancer progression, manage side effects, and prevent cancer recurrence. The clinical effectiveness of most CAM therapies remains to be definitively demonstrated, but some relevant to prostate cancer have been subjected to scientific study. These therapies are introduced in the following sections.

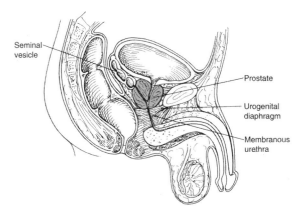

Figure 14-1 Pelvic anatomy. Note location of the prostate behind the pubis between the bladder neck (superiorly) and the urogenital diaphragm (inferiorly). Reproduced with permission from Rogers RS, Carroll PR, Tanagho E; Anatomy. In: Carroll PR, Grosseld GD, editors. Prostate Cancer. Hamilton: BC Decker Inc, 2002. p 82–92.

PREVENTION

Diet

Epidemiologic studies suggest a role for low-fat diets in prostate cancer prevention. Studies of Japanese and Chinese immigrant men in the United States show an increase in incidence compared with men in their native countries. In animal studies, low-fat diets decrease tumor growth. Data from case-control and prospective studies are mixed. Some demonstrate a direct association between increased saturated and monounsaturated fat and increased risk of prostate cancer, while others find no relationship. In a cohort study of more than 58,000 men, prostate cancer risk was not associated with the intake of total fat, total saturated fatty acids, or total trans-unsaturated fatty acids in general, although lower risk was weakly associated with increased intake of linolenic acid.

Although the role of low-fat, high-vegetable and -fruit diets in prostate cancer prevention is not fully established, such diets reduce cardiovascular risk and offer other health benefits.

Soy

Soy contains isoflavones, including the phytoestrogens genistein and daidzein. Genistein and daidzein are selective estrogen receptor modulators (SERMs). In vitro studies indicate that genistein inhibits the growth of prostate cancer cells, apparently independent of genistein's estrogenic effects. Soy intake and serum phytoestrogen levels are higher in certain Asian populations, where lower mortality rates from prostate cancer are seen.

Prospective intervention trials evaluating the role of soy product in the prevention of primary prostate cancer are lacking. Most prospective trials were done in men diagnosed with or who had been treated for prostate cancer. These studies are discussed below. Although preventive value in prostate cancer is not yet established, consumption of a moderate amount of soy protein can be beneficial, especially to the cardiovascular system.

Vitamin E

Vitamin E includes tocopherols and tocotrienols, each having four subtypes (alpha, beta, gamma, and delta). They are potent free radical scavengers and antioxidants. Recent research revealed other functions unrelated to its antioxidant activity, such as inhibition of protein kinase C, 5-lipoxygenase, cell proliferation, platelet aggregation, and monocyte adhesion.

Vitamin E inhibits the growth of prostate cancer cells in vitro at a concentration that may be achieved with oral supplementation and enhances the cytotoxic effects of Adriamycin in human prostate cancer cell lines. However, it had no effect on hyperplasia or carcinoma in a prostate cancer model in rats.

Several large clinical trials investigated the role of vitamin E in cardiovascular disease and cancer. In the Finnish Alpha-Tocopherol, Beta-Carotene (ATBC) Cancer Prevention Trial originally designed to study lung cancer, daily alpha-tocopherol was associated with a 32% reduction in incidence and a 41% decrease in mortality of prostate cancer. The Selenium and Vitamin E Cancer Prevention Trial (SELECT), a randomized, placebo-controlled, double-blind phase III prostate cancer prevention trial of 32,400 men, is underway to test the preventive efficacy of selenium and vitamin E. Final results are anticipated in 2013.

Oral vitamin E is well tolerated and appears to be relatively safe. High-dosage ($\geq$ 400 IU/d) vitamin E should not be taken for long periods of time or by those with cardiovascular risk factors. In patients with vitamin K deficiency caused by malabsorption or anticoagulant therapy, however, oral intake of high levels of vitamin E exacerbated the blood coagulation defect.

Selenium

Dietary selenium intake and serum selenium level correlate inversely with cancer risk. Selenium is a trace element required for the activity of the antioxidant enzyme glutathione peroxidase, which protects cell membranes from damage caused by the peroxidation of lipids. How selenium exercises its biologic activity remains unclear. Proposed mechanisms include interaction with redox pathways, inhibition of cell growth, induction of apoptosis, interference with cell cycle, and alteration of carcinogen metabolism.

In a multicenter, randomized, placebo-controlled study of 1,312 patients with a history of non-melanoma skin cancer (the Nutritional Prevention of Skin Cancer trial), daily intake of 200 µg of selenium lowered the incidence of prostate cancer by two-thirds. The incidence of lung and colorectal cancers also was reduced. There was no sig-

Table 14-1

FOODS RICH IN SELENIUM

Food	Micrograms (µg)
Dried Brazil nuts, unblanched, 1 ounce	544
Light tuna, canned in oil, drained, 3 ounces	63
Cooked beef, $3\frac{1}{2}$ ounces	35
Spaghetti with meat sauce, frozen entrée, 1 serving	34
Cooked cod, 3 ounces	32
Roasted turkey, light meat, $3\frac{1}{2}$ ounces	32

Reproduced from the National Institutes of Health Office of Dietary Supplements.
Daily Value for selenium is 70 µg.

nificant effect on other cancers. In the Health Professionals Follow-Up Study (HPFS), higher selenium levels were associated with reduced risk of advanced prostate cancer. The association became stronger with additional controls for family history of prostate cancer, body mass index, calcium intake, lycopene and saturated fat intake, vasectomy, and geographical region. The large-scale prostate cancer prevention trial noted above, the SELECT trial, is underway.

At the tested dose of 200 µg per day, selenium was found safe. At more than 1,000 µg per day, chronic ingestion of selenium can cause selenosis. The Institute of Medicine set a tolerable upper intake at 400 µg of selenium per day.

Plants that grow in selenium-rich soil or animals that eat such plants are good sources of dietary selenium. One ounce of Brazil nuts contains 544 µg of selenium, while 3 ounces of canned tuna contain about 63 µg of selenium. In summary, there is evidence supporting the potential of selenium in prostate cancer prevention. A definitive trial is ongoing.

Lycopene and Tomato

Lycopene is a natural pigment found in tomato, watermelon, guava, rose hip, and pink grapefruit. It is classified as a nonprovitamin A carotenoid. Epidemiologic studies suggest an inverse relationship between lycopene consumption and risk of cancer, particularly lung, prostate, and stomach. In a prospective study of male health professionals, the HPFS, frequent tomato or lycopene intake was associated with a reduced risk of prostate cancer. Intake of tomato sauce, in which lycopene is more bioavailable, was associated with an even greater reduction in prostate cancer risk, especially for extraprostatic cancers. The associations persisted even when fruit and vegetable consumption and olive oil use (a marker for Mediterranean diet) were controlled.

DURING TREATMENT

Soy

Because of its association with lower rate of prostate cancer in epidemiology studies, soy products have been studied in prostate cancer patients for their potential therapeutic value. Early stage prostate cancer patients undergoing "watchful waiting" without receiving active treatment appear to benefit from soy product intake.

In an open-label pilot study, genistein-rich soy extract was tested in 62 prostate cancer patients who had been treated with radical prostatectomy, radiotherapy, or both, hormonal therapy, or active surveillance ("watchful waiting"). None of the patients had a complete response, 17% had a partial response, 15% had stable prostate-specific antigen (PSA) levels, and 67% had progression. The active surveillance group had the best response. The data suggest that soy extract alone does not appear to be an effective treatment for prostate cancer in general. But it does lower PSA in some patients, as up to 60% of those undergoing watchful waiting showed no rise or a decline in PSA levels.

This effect in early-stage disease is confirmed by findings from another study. In a randomized controlled trial of 75 prostate cancer patients, soy isoflavone supplementation or placebo was given for 12 weeks. Changes in PSA and steroid hormones were analyzed at baseline and postintervention. Both PSA and serum free testosterone were reduced more frequently in the isoflavone group (69 and 61% respectively) than the placebo group (55 and 33%). The data suggest that supplementing early-stage prostate cancer patients with soy isoflavones, even in a study of short duration, altered surrogate markers of proliferation, although the effect is moderate.

Another randomized, prospective trial enrolled men with clinically localized prostate cancer who had selected "watchful waiting" as primary therapy. A low-fat, soy-supplemented vegan diet along with other lifestyle changes was initiated and PSA and endorectal magnetic resonance imaging data collected. Prevention of cancer recurrence by soy protein is also being studied in post–radical prostatectomy patients. These men, with PSA failure indicative of recurrence or at high risk for recurrence, were started on soy protein powder and followed for PSA failure rate and time-to-PSA failure. The results from the above two studies are pending.

Selenium

Selenium is being tested not only for primary prevention of prostate cancer, but also for inhibition of disease progression in men diagnosed with prostate cancer. Several trials are ongoing evaluating the chemopreventive effect of selenized yeast in patients with various phases of prostate cancer. The study populations are men suspected to have prostate cancer but biopsy-negative; men with high-grade prostatic intraepithelial neoplasia; men scheduled for prostatectomy; and men who elected the "watchful waiting" approach. This study is ongoing.

Lycopene

Lycopene was tested in a phase II randomized trial for its activity against prostate cancer cells prior to radical prostatectomy. Twenty-six patients were given 15 mg of lycopene twice daily or no supplement for 3 weeks prior to surgery. Statistically significant favorable findings were observed in the lycopene arm in terms of clear surgical margins and diffuse high-grade intraepithelial neoplasia. PSA decreased by 18% in the lycopene group but increased by 14% in the control group, although the difference was not statistically significant. The findings are encouraging, but the small sample size precludes a generalizable conclusion.

Polysaccharides

Another class of dietary supplements tested in prostate cancer patients is polysaccharide. The effect of polysaccharide is believed to be mediated through the immune system, as laboratory and animal studies showed activation of macrophages, natural killer cells, and granulocytes.

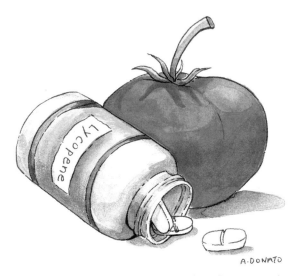

A. DONATO

Figure 14-2 Lycopene is an antioxidant that can benefit cancer patients.

Some patients may ask about a product called Genistein-Combined Polysaccharide (GCP), a fermentation product of soy extract and basidiomycete mycelia, for its purported effects on prostate cancer. The available data on this product are currently limited to in vitro and in vivo animal models. No clinical trial data is published at this point. Another polysaccharide product from a shiitake mushroom extract (SME) was tested in an uncontrolled study and found ineffective. Only 7% of the patients had stable disease after taking SME for 6 months; the rest had progression of disease. These findings compare unfavorably to the findings from the genistein-rich soy extract study conducted by the same group.

PC SPES

An herbal formulation, PC SPES received much publicity in the early 2000s as treatment for prostate cancer. At one point, approximately 10,000 patients were using PC SPES, with or without medical supervision, because it is available as a dietary supplement. PC is for "prostate cancer" and SPES comes from Latin for "hope."

Although its exact mechanism of action is unclear, the constituents have been shown to stimulate natural killer cells, inhibit growth of cancer cell lines, and bind to estrogen receptors and inhibit 5α-reductase in preclinical studies.

PC SPES consists of eight herbs: chrysanthemum, dyer's woad, Chinese licorice, reishi mushroom, pseudoginseng, rabdosia, saw palmetto, and skullcap.

Four small clinical studies demonstrated that patients with androgen-dependent or -independent prostate cancer had lower PSA levels following PC SPES treatment. Patients who progressed after chemotherapy or ketoconazole treatment, a difficult-to-treat population, still responded to PC SPES. Toxicities in those trials were similar to those expected from estrogen treatment, including gynecomastia (common), loss of libido, and venous thrombosis (uncommon).

Unfortunately, despite promising clinical activity against prostate cancer, contamination with undeclared synthetic drugs rendered this product unavailable to patients. Variable degree of contamination with indomethacin, warfarin, and diethylstilbestrol (DES) was found in several lots of PC SPES. In 2002, the U.S. Food and Drug Administration (FDA) warned consumers to stop using PC SPES, and the manufacturer (BotanicLab, Brea, CA) recalled the product and went out of business.

A recent trial compared PC SPES with DES head-to-head in 90 androgen-insensitive prostate cancer patients. In this prospective, multicenter, randomized phase II trial, decline of PSA, median response duration, and median time to progression all were superior in the PC SPES group. DES was detected in several lots of PC-SPES, the amount ranging from 0.01 to 3.1% of the dose used in the DES arm. Apparently, the clinical activity observed cannot be attributed entirely to the DES contaminant. The studies of PC SPES serve as a good example to illustrate the promise, the problems, the complexity, and the necessity of conducting rigorous scientific research of herbal products.

AFTER TREATMENT

Pelvic Symptoms

Pelvic surgery and radiation are associated with several long-term sequelae, including chronic pelvic pain, urinary incontinence, and sexual dysfunction. Complementary therapies have been explored to treat these symptoms.

A small acupuncture study was conducted in men suffering from noninflammatory chronic pelvic pain syndrome with intrapelvic venous congestion. Pain and quality of life scores improved significantly from the baseline. The maximum width of the sonolucent zone 1 week after the fifth treatment also decreased significantly when compared with baseline. Intrapelvic venous congestion was also improved.

Mind–body techniques have been explored for their potential to reduce urinary incontinence after prostatectomy. The combination of pelvic muscle exercise (PME) and biofeedback reduced the episodes, frequency, and ounces of urine lost by urinary incontinence compared with no intervention. However, differences were not statistically significant. Another study compared electromyographic biofeedback versus verbal instructions as a learning tool during pelvic muscle exercises. No significant differences between the two interventions were found.

Sexual Dysfunction

Prostate cancer patients can develop sexual dysfunction such as lack of libido and impotence from nerve damage during surgery or androgen ablation therapy. Several complementary therapies have been studied for these problems. These are discussed in more detail in Chapter 18.

Vasomotor Symptoms

Estrogen or androgen ablation can produce vasomotor symptoms (hot flashes). A few uncontrolled studies investigated acupuncture to treat these symptoms. Acupuncture was shown to attenuate tamoxifen-related hot flashes in breast cancer patients in uncontrolled studies. In prostate cancer, a small, uncontrolled study was conducted in men with vasomotor symptoms due to castration therapy. A substantial decrease in the number of hot flashes was observed in these patients. The lack of a control group and the small sample size preclude any conclusion. Several controlled trials are underway.

Osteoporosis

Hormonal therapy of prostate cancer increases the risk of osteoporosis. Because the stimulation of cancer cells with phytoestrogens is not a concern in prostate cancer, supplementation with soy products in men is less problematic (see Chapter 11).

Vitamin D supplementation may have additional benefits besides preventing osteoporosis in prostate cancer patients. Calcitrol can slow the rate of increase in PSA level in early recurrent prostate cancer. In a phase I trial of a vitamin D analogue in 25 patients with advanced hormone-refractory prostate cancer, two patients showed evidence of a partial response, and five others achieved disease stabilization for more than 6 months. A small phase II study found vitamin D deficiency in a significant percentage of patients, and vitamin D supplementation led to some improvement in metastatic prostate cancer bone pain.

READINGS AND RESOURCES

1. The Alpha-Tocopherol, Beta Carotene Cancer Prevention Study Group. The effect of vitamin E and beta carotene on the incidence of lung cancer and other cancers in male smokers. N Engl J Med 1994;330:1029–35.
2. Clark LC, Combs GF Jr, Turnbull BW, et al. Effects of selenium supplementation for cancer prevention in patients with carcinoma of the skin. A randomized controlled trial. Nutritional Prevention of Cancer Study Group. JAMA 1996;276:1957–63.
3. Oh WK, Kantoff PW, Weinberg V, et al. Prospective, multicenter, randomized phase II trial of the herbal supplement, PC-SPES, and diethylstilbestrol in patients with androgen-independent prostate cancer. J Clin Oncol. 2004 Sep 15;22(18):3705-12. Epub 2004 Aug 02.

Part III

COMPLEMENTARY THERAPIES BY THE SYMPTOMS THEY TREAT

15

Complementary Therapies for Cancer Pain

Cancer patients with difficult-to-control pain are a heterogeneous group, most often suffering from chronic pain caused directly by tumor invasion or treatment, such as chemotherapy-induced mucositis. They also may experience acute pain, such as that following surgery or procedures. Mastectomy and other pain syndromes are unique to cancer, and pain in terminal stages of disease has its own characteristics and special issues.

Cancer pain occurs in the context of a potentially deadly disease, complex and often difficult treatment, and emotional, spiritual, and social challenges. It is not surprising that pain typically is feared by cancer patients more than any other symptom, sometimes even more than the disease itself.

- Each year about nine million cancer patients worldwide report moderate to severe pain 50% of the time.
- Thirty percent of newly diagnosed cancer patients and 70 to 90% of patients with far advanced disease suffer significant pain.
- Pain remains inadequately treated despite substantial progress in pain management.
- No patient should be left to suffer.

Physicians' less-than-ideal training in pain management, plus opioid and legal concerns, may contribute to this problem. Specificity theory (pain seen as a simple pathophysiologic link of events initiated by and proportionate to tissue injury) continues to dominate much medical thinking despite having been proven incorrect. Many physicians today continue to operate within this faulty paradigm, which contains no place for the role of emotions and other modulating factors. Excessive reliance on interrupting "the pain chain" with pharmacologic or surgical interventions has led to the development of many medications and elegant pain procedures, but it still leaves millions of patients suffering in pain.

Pharmacologic interventions, helpful though they are, are not devoid of side effects. This is a particular problem for cancer patients requiring long-term pharmacologic pain management, often forcing them to choose living in pain or living with undesirable side effects. Interventional approaches, while successful and appropriate in selected patients, are not applicable to the majority of chronic pain sufferers.

A new era in pain research, initiated by Melzack's gate theory, led to new definitions of pain such as that coined by the International Association for the Study of Pain. Pain is now defined as "an unpleasant sensory and emotional experience associated with actual or potential tissue damage, or described in terms of such damage." This definition views pain as inseparable from emotions and meaning and not necessarily related to tissue injury. Importantly, degree of pain is now understood as "what the patient says it is."

> **Pain is an unpleasant sensory and emotional experience associated with actual or potential tissue damage or described in terms of such damage.**

Patients with chronic pain are heavy users of complementary therapies. These modalities work through direct analgesic effects (eg, acupuncture via opioidergic activity), by action similar to nonsteroidal anti-inflammatory drugs (NSAIDs) (eg, anti-inflammatory herbs), and by distraction, to affect pain perception, assist relaxation, improve sleep, or reduce comorbid symptoms such as nausea, vomiting, anxiety, or depressed mood. Often complementary therapies used alone successfully treat mild pain. When pain is more severe, they may enable reduction in pain medication dosage, thereby decreasing side effects, and they may work synergistically with a pain regimen, improving its effectiveness.

WORLD HEALTH ORGANIZATION THREE-STEP "LADDER" FOR CANCER PAIN RELIEF

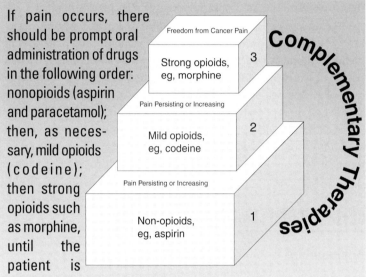

If pain occurs, there should be prompt oral administration of drugs in the following order: nonopioids (aspirin and paracetamol); then, as necessary, mild opioids (codeine); then strong opioids such as morphine, until the patient is free of pain. To calm fears and anxiety, additional drugs— "adjuvants"—should be used. To maintain freedom from pain, drugs should be given "by the clock," that is every 3–6 hours, rather than "on demand." This three-step approach of administering the right drug in the right dose at the right time is inexpensive and 80 to 90% effective. Surgical intervention on appropriate nerves may provide further pain relief if drugs are not wholly effective.

THE INTEGRATIVE APPROACH TO PAIN MANAGEMENT

Although the mechanism of action of many complementary therapies remains to be determined and evidence from randomized trials scarce, this should not discourage the incorporation of safe therapies in pain treatment plans. Applying the basic World Health Organization (WHO) analgesic ladder for cancer pain management, complementary therapies could be added to each step to provide a balance between safety and effectiveness and to encourage patient input and preference.

Most complementary interventions may safely be used early in treatment, at step 1, alone or in combination with medication, and continued as pain increases as they may act synergistically with other therapies. The optimal complementary therapy applied may well change as a function of disease progression and evolving patient needs. Acupuncture alone may be appropriate for mild pain and may be used adjunctively for patients on high doses of opioids or whose pain has neuropathic components. Patient-controlled techniques, such as meditation or self-hypnosis, are very helpful. Especially when taught to patients early in the course of disease, these interventions serve patients well throughout the process. Yoga may be used for ambulatory patients with relatively functional musculoskeletal systems, but its breathing techniques will be helpful throughout the course of disease.

SPECIFIC COMPLEMENTARY THERAPIES

Acupuncture

Acupuncture has been increasingly recognized over the past decade as an important intervention for pain relief. It can be effective regardless of the etiology of pain and potentially may be tried in many clinical situations. Modern research suggests that acupuncture analgesia is based on its opioidergic activities as well as its influence on neurotransmitters such as serotonin, catecholamines, and γ-aminobutyric acid (GABA). Functional magnetic resonance imaging (fMRI) studies show that acupuncture may activate the pain inhibiting descending pathways and deactivate areas of brain involved in pain perception.

Clinical trials conducted to date have evaluated acupuncture for multiple pain scenarios, including acute pain (procedural, postoperative), chronic musculoskeletal pain, headaches, facial and dental pain, and pain related to neuropathy in human immunodeficiency virus (HIV). Strong evidence supporting the analgesic effects of acupuncture is seen in dental pain research. In 2003, the first well designed randomized controlled trial of auricular acupuncture for chronic, neuropathic pain in breast and other cancer patients was conducted, indicating its effectiveness both with and without pharmacologic analgesia.

Severe complications related to acupuncture (eg, pneumothorax, infections secondary to improper handling of needles) although reported are extremely rare in the hands of experienced practitioners. It seems prudent to avoid acupuncture treatment in thrombocytopenic patients and for those on chronic anticoagulant therapy.

The benefits of acupuncture may stem not only from its analgesic effects, but also because it decreases nausea and fatigue and induces general relaxation. The effectiveness of acupuncture in animals and infants suggests that the effects of acupuncture are primarily physiologic and well beyond placebo benefit. It is essential to refer patients to carefully screened and qualified practitioners. Some insurance carriers cover acupuncture therapy for pain. Acupuncture is detailed in Chapter 8.

Massage

Massage belongs to a group of therapies commonly described as manipulative or body-based interventions (see Chapter 9). Massage therapy encompasses several types, but all include hands-on manipulation of muscles and soft tissue to prevent and alleviate discomfort, muscle spasm, and pain. Touch may range from extremely light to deeper, depending on the patient's clinical status. The multiple physiologic effects of massage include enhanced immune function as measured by increased levels of natural killer cells, decreased cortisol and epinephrine, and improved blood and lymph circulation.

The pain-ameliorating properties of therapeutic massage appear to result from the depletion of substance P and elevated production of endorphins. Massage therapy also modifies the transmission of impulses at the spinal cord level. At the brain level, massage seems to improve cognition, reduce stress, and help with sleep, all of which have significant roles in pain perception. A few studies evaluated massage specifically in patients with cancer. In one, massage was shown to be effective as a short-term intervention. Another study showed that massage therapy significantly reduced a range of symptoms, including pain, fatigue, anxiety, and depression, for at least 48 hours.

Most training programs in therapeutic massage have abandoned the antiquated and incorrect belief that massage therapy can "spread the cancer." Training programs in therapeutic massage for cancer patients teach licensed massage therapists to work safely and most effectively with cancer patients. Some obvious lessons include application of gentle, light-touch massage in patients with bone and vertebral metastases or significant osteoporosis, and avoidance of ports and sites with malignant lesions.

Chiropractic Manipulation

Chiropractic spinal manipulation is utilized for treatment of non-malignant pain, mostly musculoskeletal lower back pain. Chiropractic focuses on the relationship between bodily structure and the function of nervous system and the manipulation of bones and joints to restore health. Evidence does not support chiropractic manipulation for cancer patients. Major cancer centers view it as neither safe nor effective and warn against its use.

Dietary Supplements

Many dietary supplements (see Chapter 6), such as S-adenosyl-L-methionine (SAMe), methylsulfonylmethane (MSM), glucosamine, chondroitin, and turmeric, have been used empirically to treat musculoskeletal pain (chronic lower back pain, fibromyalgia) and arthritic conditions. Glucosamine appear to be beneficial for patients with osteoarthritis, but its effectiveness and safety in cancer-related pain has not been evaluated. Cancer patients may suffer from pain related to osteoarthritis, and glucosamine could ameliorate such pain. However, potential interactions between dietary supplements and use of chemotherapeutic agents (see Chapter 4) render supplement use by cancer patients problematic. Patients under active treatment should discuss use of those therapies with their oncologists before using them.

Capsaicin

Capsaicin, from capsicum hot pepper, is commonly used as a spice and also in topical preparations. It depletes local stores of substance P, which is involved in the transmission of pain impulses from peripheral nerves to spinal column. It has been used to treat postherpetic neuralgia and diabetic neuropathy. When applied for the first time it actually increases pain sensation because it activates sensory neurons, which some patients find difficult to tolerate. Analgesic effects occur with repeated applications.

Herbal Remedies

Several herbal products (see Chapters 4 and 6) have anti-inflammatory properties; *Boswellia serrata*, a well known example, works by inhibiting the production of prostaglandins. Thus, its mechanism of action is very similar to that of NSAIDs. It seems unnecessary and impractical, however, to use herbs with anti-inflammatory properties instead of NSAIDs, which are indicated for mild cancer pain and for adjunctive treatment of metastatic bone pain. Chinese herbs with analgesic and sedating effects, such as *Corydalis yanhusuo*, are used by practitioners of traditional Chinese medicine to treat pain. These have not yet been studied in cancer patients, and their use generally is not advised.

Mind–Body Therapy

Mind–body therapies (see Chapter 7) include techniques such as hypnosis, biofeedback, guided imagery, cognitive behavior therapies, and meditation. The relaxation response, a common denominator for many meditation techniques, and autogenic training produce biological effects such as decreased secretion of stress hormones and reduced oxygen consumption. The mechanism by which these therapies work may be via activation of neurotransmitters, such as serotonin and catecholamines, which influence perception of pain.

That pain perception can be modulated by one's attitudes and beliefs, which in turn can be altered by mind–body therapies, has gained increasing acceptance in recent years. Placebo analgesia, where mere belief that one is receiving an effective treatment can reduce pain, is a special situation that illustrates this phenomenon well. Researchers at the University of Michigan demonstrated that placebos reduced fMRI blood oxygen level–dependent signals in pain-sensitive brain regions including thalamus, insula, anterior cingulate cortex, and somatosensory cortex, confirming that placebos did alter the experience of pain and that pain was reversible using the μ-opioid antagonist naloxone.

Biofeedback

Biofeedback is effective primarily for nonmalignant pain such as tension headaches.

Hypnosis

The effects of pain management come in part from reprogramming the brain's response to messages from the body. Hypnotic suggestion for analgesia accomplishes this not through endorphin activation, but instead via three general mechanisms: spinal cord antinociceptive mechanisms; brain mechanisms that prevent awareness of pain once nociception has reached higher centers; and by modulating affect dimensions, possibly through the reinterpretation of meanings associated with painful sensations. A National Institutes of Health (NIH) panel strongly recommends the use of hypnosis for cancer pain. It should be more widely applied for this purpose.

Movement Therapy

Movement therapies such as yoga or tai chi are part of mainstream exercise and are widely available to the public in health clubs and elsewhere. Tai chi reduced pain and joint dysfunction from osteoarthritis in a randomized study. Yoga improves sleep quality, latency, and duration in cancer patients, although cancer pain has not yet been subjected to study. These gentle forms of exercise also incorporate breath control and meditation, mind–body components that can be helpful in combating pain. Yoga classes offered at cancer centers take patients' clinical status into account and avoid extreme postures.

Energy Therapy

Energy therapies such as Reiki or "healing touch" are popular with many patients. Reiki stems from traditional Japanese practice; healing touch comes from the nursing tradition. Both are based on ancient understanding that restoration of health requires removing "blockages" in hypothesized "energy fields" (see Chapter 2). Today's practice involves removing purported blockages with practitioners' hands. Although research does not support any component of energy field theory or practice, most patients anecdotally report a sense of deep relaxation following this practice. Such a state is helpful in the management of pain. These approaches tap the spiritual realm, which plays a significant role for many patients, especially as death approaches.

Diet

Patients rarely look to diet for pain relief. By extrapolating data from rheumatoid arthritis studies, however, some dietary modifications might be beneficial. Increased consumption of foods rich in certain essential fatty acids (EFA), may help relieve pain by decreasing or altering production of proinflammatory series 2 prostaglandins and leukotrienes. Omega-3 fatty acids, primarily alpha-linolenic acid (ALA), are found in fish, flaxseed, nuts, and seeds. Omega-6 fatty acids, of which linoleic acid (LA) is primary, come from corn, safflower, and soybean cooking oils. EFA, like vitamins, are not synthesized by the body and require dietary intake. The composition of body membranes, specifically the ratio between omega-3 and omega-6 fatty acids, affects production of various eicosanoids. Diets rich in omega-6 fatty acids enhance the production of inflammatory prostaglandins. Therefore, elimination of polyunsaturated oils (safflower, corn), minimizing intake of partially hydrogenated oils, and increasing omega-3 fatty acids consumption with oily fish, flax seed, and walnuts may help relieve pain.

Supplementation with fish oil has been shown to improve nerve conduction velocity, and preliminary studies suggest it may help treat and prevent diabetic neuropathy. Thus it may have a future role in treating cancer-related neuropathic pain.

There is interest in using EFA for cancer-related conditions such as cachexia, but its pain-reducing properties in cancer have not been evaluated. This diet modification seems very safe and may have additional benefits for cancer patients. Consuming large doses of omega-3 fatty acids decreases clotting tendency by lowering platelet aggregation and fibrinogen levels and increasing synthesis of prostaglandin I3. Because many cancer patients are in a hypercoagulable state, these effects may be beneficial. For patients on anticoagulants, this type of diet is likely to have synergistic anticoagulant effects.

CLINICAL APPLICATIONS

Untreated or poorly controlled pain has devastating effects and leads to despair. Today's cancer care is multidisciplinary and includes psychologists, social workers, clergy, hospice workers, pain and palliative care specialists, and others in addition to primary oncologists.

Today's supportive care, including complementary therapies, extends a long tradition in oncology. It is important for physicians to consider complementary modalities as part of pain management. Therapies that have low side effect profiles may be adopted more readily; those that are potentially more harmful require solid evidence prior to use. Weighing the risk-benefit ratio will assist provision of responsible, evidence-based, patient-centered advice. Complementary therapies often provide the human touch sometimes diminished in an increasingly busy and high-tech world. The ultimate benefit they may bring is to empower patients and provide comfort to the patient and family.

READINGS AND RESOURCES

1. Cassileth BR, Deng G. Complementary and alternative therapies for cancer. The Oncologist 2004;9:80–9.
2. Kaptchuk TJ. Acupuncture: theory, efficacy and practice. Ann Intern Med 2002;136:374–83.
3. National Institutes of Health (NIH). Integrated approach to the management of pain. NIH Consensus Statement. Vol. 6, No. 3; May 19–21, 1986. Available at: http://consensus.nih.gov/cons/055/055_intro.htm (accessed March 10, 2005).
4. National Institutes of Health (NIH). NIH state-of-the-science conference statement on symptom management in cancer: pain, depression and fatigue. July 15–17, 2002. Available at: http://odp.od.nih.gov/consensus/ta/022/022_intro.htm (accessed March 10, 2005).
5. Pan CX, Morrison RS, Ness J, et al. Complementary and alternative medicine in the management of pain, dyspnea and nausea and vomiting near end the end of life: a systematic review. J Pain Sympt Manage 2000;20:374–87.

16

Mood Disturbance and Fatigue

MOOD DISTURBANCE

Anxiety and depression are highly prevalent in cancer patients. About one in four experience major depression at some point during their illness, with a point prevalence of 3 to 12% in early stage disease and 10 to 30% among patients with metastatic cancer. Anxiety is reported by 25 to 50% of cancer patients at any one time. A small proportion of patients will have underlying disorder predating their cancer diagnosis, but mood disorders occur commonly throughout the trajectory of major illness.

Short-term anxiety and depression are common and arguably appropriate responses to initial diagnosis or recurrence. Treatment or diagnostic procedures, such as surgery or a scan, often evoke acute anxiety. In some patients, however, mood disturbance persists well after initial adjustment and requires intervention. Depression may occur in response to treatment toxicity (eg, from interferon). Depression also may occur as a consequence of the physical side effects of disease or treatment, such as pain, fatigue, and nausea. Importantly, spiritual or existential concerns may underlie and give rise to what may be seen as mood disorder. Often underappreciated, such circumstances require intervention.

Anxiety and depression increase with advancing cancer and constitute significant burdens for end-of-life patients and families and major challenges for the oncology professionals who organize and provide their care.

Conventional management of anxiety and depression in cancer is based on psychotherapy and pharmacotherapy. Although of undoubted effectiveness, anxiety and depression are insufficiently recognized in standard oncologic care unless formal screening is implemented.

Psychiatric screening is not routinely available in most settings, and many patients are not prone to seek assistance on their own. Patients may see psychiatric diagnosis and treatment as stigmatizing or a symptom of inability to cope adequately with illness. They may decline assistance or fail to seek it, uncomfortable about categorizing themselves as "mentally ill" and unwilling to acknowledge a need for psychiatric care. Indeed the vast majority of cancer patients are not mentally ill. Rather they are suffering severe psychological stress that would benefit from assistance. It is estimated that one in three cancer patients in need of psychiatric or psychological help refuse intervention.

Helpful and appropriate intervention can take various forms, including medication, spiritual guidance, or complementary therapies. The importance of patient preference—what "feels" right and appropriate to that patient—is key. Patients who self-select complementary interventions can do so without prescription and according to their personal preference. Many complementary therapies involve self-help, which is highly valued by patients today. Others simply provide all-important comfort and a sense of peace. A basic value of these therapies is their ability to relieve many of the distressing emotional symptoms that all but inevitably accompany the diagnosis and treatment of cancer.

Massage Therapies

Massage is widely perceived as relaxing. There is now good evidence from randomized trials that massage therapy relieves anxiety in groups as varied as adolescent psychiatric patients, intensive care unit patients, elderly people in nursing homes, and children suffering post-traumatic stress disorder. Several studies have examined the effects of massage therapy on psychological endpoints in cancer patients. In a high-quality if underpowered trial, 35 inpatients undergoing autologous bone marrow transplantation were randomized to receive either up to nine 20-minute massages or standard care. Psychometric instruments were administered before, during, and after the course of treatment, including the State-Trait Anxiety Inventory, the Beck Depression Inventory, the Brief Profile of Mood States, and numerical rating scales of distress, fatigue, nausea, and pain. Massage was superior to standard care for anxiety, nausea, fatigue, and general well-being.

In another clinical trial, 87 hospitalized cancer patients were randomized to foot massage or control care on a crossover basis. A visual analogue scale of anxiety was completed immediately before and after each treatment session. Anxiety scores were significantly lower following massage, but little change followed the control procedures ($p < 0.001$).

Several randomized trials compared massage therapy with standard care versus aromatherapy oils in cancer patients. Although generally failing to show that aromatherapy oils add benefit, these trials provided clinically relevant data, indicating decreased anxiety scores in both groups receiving massage. For example, in 51 hospice patients randomized to a course of massage with or without the addition of aromatherapy oil, anxiety scores improved from approximately 30 to 20 on the Spielberger State Anxiety inventory in both groups. Another study found that anxiety and depression scores on the Hospital Anxiety and Depression Scale fell by a median of two points in the combined groups.

In a single-arm outcome study of massage, anxiety and depression were rated on a 0–10 numerical rating scale immediately before and immediately after a single massage treatment. Scores on both scales improved by approximately 50% for both outpatients and inpatients. In a subsample followed further, benefits persisted for at least the 48-hour follow-up period.

Mind–Body Therapies

A meta-analysis of 15 randomized trials assessed the effect of progressive muscle relaxation therapies in several oncology settings such as chemotherapy and bone marrow transplantation. Six studies involving a total of 274 subjects included depression as an endpoint; eight studies with 351 patients assessed anxiety. The effect size for both was statistically significant, approximately one-half a standard deviation better than for control subjects. However, because techniques involving progressive muscle relaxation induce anxiety in 17 to 31% of patients, most commonly because of intrusive thoughts, fear of losing control, and restlessness, other mind–body techniques such as meditation and hypnosis may be more useful for cancer patients.

Randomized trials have examined the effects of meditation on anxiety and depression in outpatients. In a typical study, 109 cancer patients with varying diagnoses and stages of disease were randomized to received seven weekly 90-minute meditation classes and encouraged to practice meditation at home. Mood was assessed at baseline and after the final treatment using the Profile of Mood States. Anxiety and depression scores fell by nearly 50% in the meditation group with little change in control subjects.

Examples of other randomized trials include reductions in anxiety and depression following 1-hour relaxation training sessions in women with gynecologic cancers; group support plus relaxation training decreased mood disturbance more effectively than group support alone in early stage breast cancer patients, and relaxation training and benzodiazepine (alprazolam) were comparable in relieving anxiety and depression.

Music Therapy

There has been considerable research on the effects of music on mood, especially in the acute medical setting (see Chapter 10). An early randomized trial enrolled patients hospitalized following myocardial infarction. Patients listening to music tapes reported significantly reduced anxiety scores compared with no-treatment control subjects. Similar results were found in a replication trial, using an attention control arm, suggesting that the benefits resulted from music rather than from a nonspecific effect of attention. Randomized trials also have demonstrated that recorded music reduces anxiety before or after surgical procedures.

In a study conducted in 1983, 50 hospitalized cancer patients were randomly assigned to either a live music therapy session or taped music control treatment. Patients receiving live music had significantly lower anxiety scores than those listening to tapes. In another trial, 69 autologous bone marrow transplant patients were randomized either to a course of treatment from music therapists during their inpatient stay or to standard care alone. Mood was assessed before and after music therapy (or equivalent control period) over the course of hospitalization. Anxiety scores on the Profile of Mood States fell by approximately one-half immediately following music therapy, but by only about 10% in control subjects ($p = 0.003$ for difference between groups). When measured over the course of the inpatient stay, anxiety scores were approximately 33% lower in the music therapy group ($p = 0.013$). Differences between groups were very much smaller for depression, possibly as a result of low baseline depression scores in this sample.

The effects of music therapy on acute distress associated with cancer-related procedures are less clear. Although evidence from randomized trials suggests that use of prerecorded music lowers anxiety in women awaiting breast biopsy and in patients undergoing sigmoidoscopy, trials examining music during radiation therapy for prostate cancer or during a variety of diagnostic and other procedures did not find beneficial effects for music.

The contrasting results of these studies offer several lessons. First, music may be subject to adverse classical conditioning. In the prostate cancer study, music was presented during repeated radiotherapy sessions and may have become associated with the anxiogenic stimulus. This effect would not occur during a single session of music therapy for women awaiting breast biopsy. Second, music during procedures is a distraction. This may be beneficial for some procedures (eg, sigmoidoscopy), but it is not appropriate if the patient wishes to pay attention, as may be the case in diagnostic work-ups shortly after a cancer diagnosis.

Acupuncture

Acupuncture is anecdotally described as relaxing. A few small randomized trials have reported reductions in both acute and chronic anxiety. However, no studies to date have examined the effects of acupuncture on mood in cancer patients.

Herbal Medicines

St. John's wort is of proven value for mild to moderate depression, and, more recently, for severe depression. It is at least equivalent in efficacy to tricyclic antidepressants and selective serotonin reuptake inhibitors (SSRIs), but its side effect profile is superior to both. St. John's wort induces cytochrome P-450 (CYP3A4) and therefore interacts with agents metabolized on this pathway. Reduced plasma levels of SN38, an active metabolite of irinotecan, have been reported following simultaneous use. Such metabolic interactions preclude St. John's wort for cancer patients during treatment.

Kava is a recreational drug with proven anxiolytic properties. However, it is associated with hepatotoxicity and is banned in several countries, including the United Kingdom and France. *Valerian*

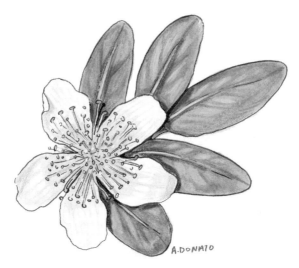

Figure 16-1 Research supports the use of St. John's wort for mild, moderate, and severe depression.

is a traditional treatment for insomnia. Several small, randomized trials indicate a mild hypnotic action. These agents can have effects similar to those of benzodiazepines.

Many plants contain psychoactive substances, and it is this property that underlies their use as recreational drugs. For St. John's wort, hypericin, and hyperforin have been separately identified as active components, and amentoflavone recently was demonstrated to be psychoactive. It is also known that different constituents have additive or synergistic effects on amine receptors in vitro, suggesting that the activity of St. John's wort cannot be ascribed to a single constituent. Kava contains kavapyrones, which has known effects on the dopaminergic system and on γ-aminobutyric acid (GABA) binding. Valerian contains a large number of potentially psychoactive substances, including the valepotriates, although the exact contribution of these constituents to valerian's hypnotic action is not yet known.

Because the content of these bioactive constituents varies considerably across supplements from different manufacturers and different lots from the same manufacturer, they may produce unpredictable effects in some individuals. It is prudent for cancer patients to refrain from using these supplements during active treatment (see Chapter 4).

Clinical Application

Integrative therapies are typically used to treat mild and subclinical anxiety and depression. It is not unusual for patients with symptoms to use integrative modalities alone to manage mild symptoms of mood disorder, forgoing other psychotherapeutic or pharmacologic intervention.

KEY ADVANTAGES OF INTEGRATIVE THERAPIES FOR MOOD DISORDER IN ONCOLOGY

- The only stigma or label attached to the recommendation or use of complementary therapies is that of proactive coping.
- Patients may themselves select therapies to which they are drawn and from which they derive comfort.
- The self-care and coping involved is deeply valued by many patients today.

SEVERE ANXIETY AND DEPRESSION

Integrative therapies have been used also as adjuncts in the treatment of more severe anxiety and depressive disorders. This is usually as part of a package of care, led by a psychiatrist, that includes psychotherapy and appropriate medication. Some therapies used by practitioners of integrative medicine, such as hypnosis, meditation, or imagery (see Chapter 7), are commonly applied by mental health professionals. Hypnosis in particular effectively reduces anxiety, including presurgery anxiety.

Fatigue

Fatigue is extremely prevalent in cancer patients, particularly those undergoing chemotherapy or radiotherapy. In a population-based survey of nearly 400 cancer patients treated with chemotherapy, 60% indicated experiencing fatigue at least once a week during the most recent chemotherapy cycle, and 70% said that fatigue interfered with their daily lives. Although most patients recover prediagnosis energy levels within a few months of completing cytotoxic therapy, a minority of patients continues to experience fatigue for months or even years.

Studies suggest that adjuvant therapy produces chronic fatigue in approximately one in eight patients. Fatigue in cancer patients is not always related to treatment. For example, the prevalence of fatigue is estimated at approximately 50% in patients with advanced cancer receiving no oncologic treatment.

Current treatment guidelines recommend identification and correction of primary factors causing fatigue, such as anemia, thyroid dysfunction, sleep disturbance, pain, and distress. When these factors are controlled, education and counseling about energy preservation, distraction, and stress management should be provided. In addition, exercise, restorative therapy, and pharmacologic intervention (psychostimulants, antidepressants, and steroids) may be used for symptomatic treatment. Several complementary modalities have been studied for the relief of fatigue. Most fatigue studies were conducted in noncancer patients, such as those with chronic fatigue syndrome or multiple sclerosis. The few representative studies on cancer-related fatigue are discussed below.

Massage Therapies

One randomized trial and one cohort study assessing the effects of massage on a variety of symptoms included the assessment of fatigue. In a trial of 33 patients undergoing autologous bone marrow transplant, fatigue was measured before and after each of three massages or equivalent periods of "quiet time." Post-treatment fatigue scores were lower in the massage group by about 1.5 points on a 0–10 scale. Data from a cohort study of patients receiving massage were analyzed for patients who reported at least moderate distress for fatigue, depression, pain, or anxiety) at baseline (defined as a score of 4 or above). Symptom scores were reduced by 43% from a mean baseline of 6.6 in 819 patients.

Music Therapy

In a trial of music therapy for overall mood disturbance in patients undergoing autologous bone marrow transplant, results were reported for each subscale of the Profile of Mood States, allowing evaluation of the effects of music on fatigue independent of its effects on other mood states. Sixty-nine patients were randomized to receive either a course of treatments from music therapists during their inpatient stay or to standard care alone. Patients completed the Profile of Mood States before and after each music therapy session (or equivalent control period) and over the course of hospitalization. Fatigue scores on the Profile of Mood States improved by about one-third immediately following music therapy but only by about 5% in control subjects (p = 0.02). When measured over the course of the inpatient stay, fatigue scores were approximately 25% lower in the music therapy group (p = 0.03).

Acupuncture

In a single-arm, Phase II trial, 39 nonanemic cancer patients with chronic postchemotherapy fatigue (mean duration close to 2 years) received six to eight acupuncture treatments over the course of 4 to 6 weeks. Fatigue was assessed using the Brief Fatigue Inventory at baseline and at the end of treatment. Mean improvement in fatigue scores following treatment was 31% in the 31 patients who completed the trial. Improvement was found to be negatively correlated with age; mean improvement in patients aged under 65 years was close to 38%. Among the 14 patients with severe fatigue at baseline, 11 (79%) reported nonsevere fatigue scores after treatment. The effect of acupuncture treatment for cancer-related fatigue requires confirmation in a controlled trial.

Mind–Body Therapies

Although definitive trials showing effectiveness have not yet been conducted, the National Comprehensive Cancer Network (NCCN) recommends relaxation techniques, restorative therapy such as spiritual activity and meditation, and sleep therapy as nonpharmacologic interventions for stress management. These therapies should be considered for fatigue as well. They are safe and associated with other quality of life benefits.

Tibetan yoga was evaluated in a randomized study of 39 lymphoma patients. The intervention was yoga practices of Tsa lung and Trul khor, which incorporate controlled breathing and visualization, mindfulness techniques, and low-impact postures. Although fatigue was not a primary endpoint, it was included in the outcome measures. When compared with wait-list control subjects, no significant difference was observed in fatigue, anxiety, or depression, but significant improvement was seen for sleep quality, latency, and duration, and the use of sleep medication was reduced. In another randomized wait-list control study, mindfulness-meditation did not significantly reduce the fatigue subscale on the Profile of Mood States. Significant improvement of other mood subscales, however, was reported.

Nutrition and Dietary Supplements

Cancer and cancer treatment can lead to decreased nutrition intake. Changes in taste and appetite, along with nausea alteration of gut anatomy, can contribute to lower intake and absorption. Adequate protein and caloric intake is important. Some diet regimens are promoted as alternative cancer treatments. Typically restrictive, these limit the intake of certain foods or food categories (see Chapter 5). Special diet regimens that do not include all major food groups can lead to malnourishment, and malnourishment can cause fatigue.

Numerous dietary supplements are promoted as energy boosters, but few have been evaluated to determine the merits of such claims (see Chapter 6). The herb ginseng is used in East Asia as an energy booster. Three species of plants are commonly called ginseng: Siberian ginseng (*Eleutherococcus senticosus*), Asian ginseng (*Panax ginseng*, see Figure 16-1), and American ginseng (*Panax quinquefolius*). A major constituent, ginsenosides, has demonstrated central nervous system (CNS) stimulatory activity. Because other CNS stimulants, such as methylphenidate and modafinil, are used off label by physicians to treat cancer-related fatigue, it is plausible that ginseng may reduce fatigue. A randomized placebo-controlled trial was conducted to test Siberian ginseng for chronic fatigue in noncancer patients. No statistically significant difference between the groups was found. However, the treatment was effective in patients with less severe fatigue. Further research would be of value.

Supplementation of vitamin B_{12} and folic acid to pemetrexed treatment of mesothelioma reduced the incidence of chemotherapy-related fatigue almost by one-half in a randomized trial of 64 patients. In a single-arm trial of 44 patients with low plasma carnitine levels undergoing cisplatin treatment, supplementation with L-carnitine restored plasma levels and ameliorated fatigue with a significant increase in mean Functional Assessment of Cancer Therapy – Fatigue scores (from 19.7 to 34.9). Supplementation with essential fatty acids

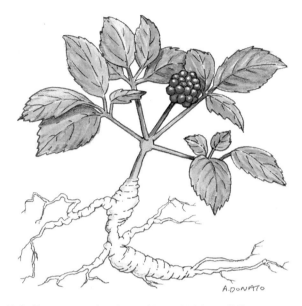

Figure 16-2 Ginseng contains ginsenoides, which have CNS stimulatory activity

(linoleic, gamma-linolenic, eicosapentaenoic, and docosahexaenoic acids) may reduce postviral fatigue. A putative mechanism is their anti-inflammatory activity, as evidence suggests that proinflammatory cytokines may be the cause of cancer-related fatigue.

Clinical Application

Fatigue in cancer patients remains inadequately treated, primarily because of the lack of effective therapies other than correction of anemia. Other mainstream interventions have their own limitations. Patients may not be compliant with exercise programs. Psychostimulants still are under investigation and are associated with side effects. Many patients therefore try to deal with fatigue on their own, and many are attracted to the unwarranted claims of "alternative" therapies (see Chapter 19).

The current state of science is that complementary therapies have not been shown to be reliably effective against cancer-related fatigue, although some evidence supports their helpfulness in selected patients. Therefore, the decision to recommend complementary therapies depends on the level of risk. Massage, mind–body therapies, and other techniques that are safe and shown to reduce other symptoms can be tried. Caution must be exercised concerning the use of dietary supplements. Those that have no adverse interactions with concurrent medications and that can correct a particular patient's dietary deficiency are acceptable. Herbal products and other supplements with potentially adverse effects (see Chapters 4 and 19) should be discouraged.

READINGS AND RESOURCES

1. Cleeland CS. Cancer-related fatigue: new directions for research. Introduction. Cancer 2001;92(6 Suppl):1657–61.
2. Ernst E, Rand JI, Stevinson C. Complementary therapies for depression: an overview. Arch Gen Psychiatry 1998;55:1026–32.
3. Mamtani R, Cimino A. A primer of complementary and alternative medicine and its relevance in the treatment of mental health problems. Psychiatr Q 2002;73:367–81.
4. Mock V, Atkinson A, Barsevick A, et al. NCCN Practice Guidelines for Cancer-Related Fatigue. Oncology (Hunting) 2000;14:151–61.

17

Gastrointestinal Symptoms

It is not unusual for patients across cancer diagnoses to experience gastrointestinal (GI) symptoms as a consequence of treatment, stress, advancing disease, or organs affected. Several complementary therapies, including acupuncture, mind–body approaches, and herbal medicines, serve well as adjunctive treatments for specific GI indications. This chapter addresses nausea and vomiting, diarrhea and constipation, xerostomia, oral mucositis and cachexia, common problems most effectively decreased by complementary modalities.

NAUSEA AND VOMITING

Nausea and vomiting tend to be closely associated with chemotherapy in the public mind. In part, this perception is a relic of cancer treatment prior to the new generation of 5-hydroxytryptamine (5-HT_3) receptor antagonist antiemetics, when three-quarters of patients on chemotherapy experienced these distressing side effects. Similarly misplaced, however, is the perception of some health professionals that, given the new antiemetics, nausea and vomiting no longer occur. In a 1983 study, cancer patients ranked vomiting and nausea as the first and second most severe side effects of chemotherapy. A replication 10 years later after the introduction of the 5-HT_3-receptor antagonists, however, showed that vomiting and nausea ranked fifth and first, respectively. The prevalence of nausea and vomiting among patients treated according to American Society of Clinical Oncology (ASCO) antiemetic guidelines is estimated at 60 to 75% and 40 to 50%, respectively.

Nausea and vomiting are also associated with radiotherapy and with end-stage disease. Almost all patients who receive high-dose total body irradiation experience emesis as do about half of those receiving conventional doses of radiation to the upper abdomen. Approximately 20% of patients with advanced cancer receiving palliative care report nausea, with a notably higher prevalence in stomach and gynecologic cancers.

Conventional management of acute chemotherapy-related nausea consists of a 5-HT$_3$-receptor antagonist such as ondansetron, along with a steroid such as dexamethasone. This has greatest efficacy in the immediate postinfusion period. Pharmacologics are only moderately beneficial against prechemotherapy ("anticipatory") nausea, which affects about one in three patients, and against low-grade nausea that persists for several days after chemotherapy (so-called "delayed nausea").

Massage Therapy

Although there is no reason to believe that tissue manipulation directly affects nausea and vomiting, massage does decrease arousal and acts as a form of distraction. Both of these benefits are valuable in treating nausea and vomiting. Two randomized trials and one cohort study assessed the effects of massage therapy on nausea and other symptoms. In a randomized, crossover study conducted in Australia, nausea scores decreased by approximately one-third following a single massage, while little or no change occurred in control subjects. A randomized trial of 33 patients undergoing autologous bone marrow transplant measured nausea before and after each of three massages or equivalent periods of "quiet time." Post-treatment nausea scores were lower in the massage group at a statistically significant level.

Both of these studies may underestimate the effects of massage on nausea because they included patients with low baseline scores. Mean baseline nausea in the Australian study, for example, was less than 2 on a 0–10 scale. In a cohort study of patients who reported at least moderate nausea at baseline, symptom scores were reduced from immediately before to immediately after treatment by approximately 50% from a mean baseline of 6.0 in 222 patients. The duration of the effects of massage against nausea are not known. Massage appears best indicated as a "well-being" treatment for patients with low-grade nausea, particularly if they are experiencing concomitant symptoms such as fatigue, anxiety, or depression.

Mind–Body Therapies

Several well-known phenomena demonstrate cognitive mediation of nausea and vomiting. Examples include vomiting related to "stage fright" and anticipatory nausea, where stimuli associated with chemotherapy, such as driving past the hospital building, themselves cause nausea. A variety of cognitive behavioral techniques have been developed to address chemotherapy nausea and vomiting, many of which include hypnosis and relaxation techniques.

Although many studies are small, the majority of randomized trials show clinically and statistically significant benefit in patients assigned to relaxation or hypnosis compared with control subjects. For example, 60 inpatients scheduled to receive multiple chemotherapy infusions were randomized to receive relaxation therapy, taped music (attention control), or standard care. Whereas approximately 80% of patients in the usual care and attention control groups experienced similar or worse vomiting at their final session compared with the prerandomization baseline, 50% of patients in the relaxation group actually improved, with statistically significant differences between the groups.

Self-managed mind–body techniques are best taught in advance so that patients can apply them when needed. Credentialed practitioners may be available to teach patients relaxation, or patients may be trained in self-hypnosis by a credentialed therapist. Also, hospital libraries may have training tapes. Not all patients will want to pursue these techniques, but others may appreciate the ability to control symptoms that mind–body training can bestow. Symptoms that are refractory or delayed and those that have a clear psychological component, such as anticipatory nausea, may also benefit from psychological management.

Acupuncture

The mechanism of acupuncture in treating emesis is not yet fully understood. However, research on acupuncture for pain has demonstrated the importance of serotonergic pathways. For example, serotonin antagonists and precursors respectively block and potentiate acupuncture analgesia in animal models. In particular, the 5-HT_3-receptor antagonist ICS 205-930 has been shown to block the analgesic effect of electroacupuncture in rabbits.

Strong evidence supports the effectiveness of acupuncture for nausea and vomiting in the surgical setting. In a meta-analysis of 26 studies involving 3,347 patients, acupuncture reduced both nausea (relative risk compared with placebo control group 0.71;95% CI 0.56–0.91; five trials) in the immediate postoperative period. These findings were robust to sensitivity analyses of study size and quality. The effects of acupuncture did not appear to persist beyond 8 hours.

A small number of pediatric studies failed to find differences between acupuncture and control treatment. Some claim that this was because of inappropriate choice of acupuncture points, and two subsequent double-blind, placebo-controlled, randomized trials indicate this may have been the case. Using acupuncture points specifically chosen for a pediatric population, these two trials included a total of 115 children. In both, rates of vomiting in the first 24 hours after surgery were approximately 20% in the acupuncture-treated patients compared with about 60% in control subjects.

In a meta-analysis of randomized trials of acupuncture for chemotherapy-related nausea and vomiting, acupuncture reduced the incidence of acute vomiting (nine trials; 1,214 patients; relative risk compared with placebo control group 0.76;95% CI 0.58–0.98 with a trend for reduction of acute nausea severity (seven trials; 895 patients; standardized mean difference 0.11; 95% CI 0.02–0.25).

Because acute nausea and vomiting are relatively well controlled in most patients, providing acupuncture routinely during chemotherapy is not warranted and would not be cost-effective. Acupuncture is more appropriate for the minority of patients who experience acute nausea and vomiting and for delayed nausea and vomiting. The primary problem for most patients is delayed, rather than acute, nausea and vomiting.

Because the antiemetic effects of acupuncture treatment appear to last only approximately 8 hours, acupuncture treatment could be arranged for later that day or for the following day near the patient's home.

Some recommend devices that provide continuing stimulation, such as the ReliefBand, a wristwatch-like device that emits a mild electrical stimulus to an acupuncture point on the wrist. However, such devices do not seem effective and have been shown to exacerbate nausea by acting as a Pavlovian conditioned stimulus for nausea.

The most appropriate role of acupuncture antiemesis in cancer chemotherapy appears to be in the treatment of severe, refractory vomiting or for severe delayed nausea, although in the latter case, it is likely that daily acupuncture treatment is required. Some clinicians recommend that patients be instructed to apply pressure to acupuncture points using their fingers. There is some evidence that this may benefit both acute and delayed nausea, and it may help patients feel more in control of their symptoms.

Herbal Medicine

Several herbs are said to have antiemetic properties. The best known is ginger, for which there is evidence of benefit from randomized trials conducted in postoperative and pregnancy-related nausea. There is also evidence that ginger is effective against cisplatin-induced emesis in the animal model. Clinical trials of herbal antiemetics in cancer patients have not been conducted. The value of herbal treatments for chemotherapy nausea and vomiting is limited by the possibility of interactions with cytotoxic therapy (see Chapter 4).

DIARRHEA AND CONSTIPATION

Constipation is a well-known side effect of opioids, particularly in the postoperative setting and among end-stage patients receiving aggressive pain management. The mechanism involved is thought to include reduction of GI motility and increased GI tone. Constipation and diarrhea may also result from chemotherapy and are among those symptoms reported by patients as most troubling. Chemotherapy causes mucosal damage to the metabolically active epithelial tissues of the GI tract, altering absorption. Chemotherapy may also cause GI side effects as a result of fluid and electrolyte imbalance.

Acute onset of diarrhea or constipation warrants evaluation to identify the underlying etiology. In chronic diarrhea or constipation where cause cannot be identified or is not subject to definitive treatment, symptomatic relief becomes the primary treatment goal. Most physicians are familiar with prescription and over-the-counter drugs used for these symptoms. Their prolonged use, however, creates unwanted side effects, and complementary therapies can be helpful in these cases.

Few methodologically sound studies have addressed the ability of integrative therapies to manage constipation and diarrhea in cancer patients. Although hypnotherapy is of proven benefit for patients without cancer who suffer from irritable bowel syndrome, application to the cancer population is unclear. Acupuncture, massage, and reflexology (foot massage) have been promoted for use in functional constipation. Although randomized trials are yet to be conducted, anecdotal reports indicate that acupuncture benefits some patients and may be worthy of pursuit.

Botanicals

TJ-14 is a Kampo botanical medicine (see Chapter 3) that incorporates various herbs used traditionally to treat GI disorders. These include ginger, Huang Lian, licorice, and skullcap. A small trial published in Japanese found that 18 of 23 patients taking TJ-14 with irinotecan experienced a good response, defined as only grade 1 diarrhea that lasted for 3 days or less. In a subsequent randomized trial of patients with non-small cell lung cancer treated with irinotecan, rates of grade 3 or 4 diarrhea were 1/18 (6%) in TJ-14-treated patients compared with 10/23 (43%) in control subjects. Although this difference is clinically and statistically significant, the trial is small, and it is possible that the beneficial effects were actually related to a metabolic interaction with the chemotherapy agent. It is plausible that TJ-14 reduced the toxicity of irinotecan by altering its metabolism or excretion or by reducing its cytotoxic effects generally. Many herbs have this effect (see Chapter 4). Appropriate studies confirming that TJ-14 does not reduce the effects of irinotecan have not been reported.

Several studies indicate that probiotics may successfully treat diarrhea and constipation, especially in irritable bowel disease. Because many cancer patients are on opioids for chronic pain or frequent antibiotics, both of which alter bowel flora, probiotics may be appropriate to try in select patients. In addition, dietary change can help control bowel problems, and patients should be encouraged to make the appropriate adjustments to their eating habits.

Xerostomia

Xerostomia, the subjective experience of extreme dry mouth, is a common side effect of radiotherapy for head and neck cancer.

Radiation-induced damage to the salivary glands can reduce salivary flow by half within a week of starting radiotherapy. Salivary function usually continues to decline for 6 to 8 months after therapy, and many patients show no recovery even at 12 months.

Xerostomia is more than an unpleasant symptom. It can have substantial impact on the patient's ability to eat and to function in employment or social situations because of its effects on speech and food consumption. Decreased salivation also can lead to dental caries, periodontal diseases, shift of oral flora, poor tolerability to dental prosthesis and inflammation, atrophy, and ulceration. In addition, salivary gland dysfunction contributes to systemic problems including loss of appetite, chronic esophagitis, gastroesophageal reflux, and sleep disruption owing to the need for frequent mouth moistening and subsequent polyuria.

Several new techniques can help reduce damage to salivary glands and preserve salivary function. These include conformal and intensity-modulated radiation therapy and administration of amifostine, a radioprotector. Current treatment of radiation-induced xerostomia includes dietary and oral hygiene and saliva substitution or stimulation of salivation by moistening agents or medications. The most effective pharmacologic treatment for xerostomia is pilocarpine. However, this medication has important drawbacks. A significant proportion of patients do not benefit from it, its effects last only a few hours, and the drug often requires 2 months or longer to achieve maximum effect. This is a particular problem because pilocarpine is associated with autonomic side effects, such as sweating.

Acupuncture

Several single-arm studies report encouraging findings for the use of acupuncture to treat radiotherapy-induced xerostomia. In a series of 50 patients, for example, a median of five acupuncture treatments over the course of a month reduced subjective xerostomia scores by 10% or more in 70% of patients. Approximately one-third of patients reported at least halving their scores. The only randomized controlled trial of acupuncture for radiotherapy-induced xerostomia was somewhat underpowered, with only 41 patients. Nonetheless, a reanalysis comparing the number of days to achieve a 0.1g/min increase in salivary flow rates between groups was published. The reported hazard ratio of 2.4 (95% CI 0.8–6.8; $p = 0.11$) indicates that acupuncture was beneficial.

ORAL MUCOSITIS

Mucositis is a complication of both radiotherapy and chemotherapy. It may result from direct cytotoxicity against the oral mucosa or from decreased ability to control minor oral infections owing to myelo-suppression. Mucositis is a particularly severe problem in high-dose therapy with stem cell support, affecting approximately three-quarters of patients. It is reportedly one of the most debilitating side effects of high-dose therapy. Pain related to mucositis can be severe enough to be a dose-limiting toxicity, particularly for regimens that combine radiation with chemotherapy.

Some evidence suggests that the severity of oral mucositis can be reduced by appropriate oral care before and during treatment. Hygienic measures to reduce the microbial load of the oral cavity are neither expensive nor toxic and are generally advised for patients scheduled to receive therapy associated with a high risk of mucositis. Mucositis may be prevented in some patients by the use of oral cryotherapy: patients suck on ice chips for about half an hour before an infusion with the aim of reducing blood flow and hence reduced transport of cytotoxic agents to the oral cavity. Neither cryothera-py nor hygienic measures such as mouthwashes are completely effec-tive against mucositis, and the mainstay of care is topical plus systemic treatment with opioids.

Botanicals

Several botanical medicines are purported to have beneficial and pro-tective effects on the skin (note, for example, the preponderance of botanical extracts in beauty products), and some popular botanicals are now incorporated into mouthwashes for the treatment of mucosi-tis. Although preliminary evidence was provocative, a mouthwash containing an extract of chamomile was not found to prevent 5-fluorouracil (5FU)–induced mucositis.

A more encouraging finding was reported for a product known as Traumeel S. Although this is often described as a homeopathic product, suggesting that it contains negligible doses of pharmaco-logically active substances (see Chapter 2), Traumeel S may be better characterized as a botanical medicine because it contains several botanical extracts, although in more dilute form than is common for botanical agents.

In a randomized, placebo-controlled trial with 30 children undergoing stem cell transplantation, patients receiving Traumeel mouthwashes reported less severe mucositis than did control subjects. The proportion of Traumeel-treated patients experiencing mucositis (~45%) was one-half that of placebo-treated control subjects (~90%). There was no effect on GI stomatitis or neutropenia, suggesting that the effect of Traumeel S is local.

Mind–Body Therapies

Mind–body therapies are widely used to treat both acute and chronic cancer-related pain, and a number of randomized trials suggest that they are effective (see Chapter 7). Some of the best evidence for mind–body therapies for acute pain comes from the stem cell transplant setting. In an early clinical trial of 67 patients undergoing high-dose therapy, oral mucositis pain was lower in a group receiving hypnotherapy as compared with patients randomized to standard care, cognitive behavior therapy, or to a "therapist contact" control group. A subsequent study confirmed that this effect was cognitively mediated: pain levels differed between groups despite similar levels of mucositis severity, as rated by an independent observer on the basis of a visual inspection.

CACHEXIA

Cachexia is prevalent among patients with end-stage disease and is commonly involved in the mode of death. Cachexia is often associated with anorexia, which can result from chemotherapy-induced nausea, and with changes in taste and smell. Anorexia may also be caused by early satiety following surgery for GI cancer, and by psychological morbidity. Yet cachexia can occur in the absence of anorexia as a result of tumor-produced factors and metabolic abnormalities.

Cachexia typically is managed by aggressive nutritional therapy. Some had suggested that dietary supplements containing essential fatty acids, such as fish oil or evening primrose oil, might be useful adjuncts to nutritional management. However, while early single-arm studies showed promising results, subsequent randomized, double-blind trials failed to show any important effects of fatty acid supplementation on appetite or weight gain. In some cases, the supplements were not well tolerated by patients.

READINGS AND RESOURCES

1. Johnstone PA, Niemtzow RC, Riffenburgh RH. Acupuncture for xerostomia: clinical update. Cancer 2002;94:1151–6.
2. Lee A, Done M. Stimulation of the wrist acupuncture point P6 for preventing postoperative nausea and vomiting. Cochrane Database Syst Rev 2004;3:CD003281.
3. Morrow GR, Morrell C. Behavioral treatment for the anticipatory nausea and vomiting induced by cancer chemotherapy. N Engl J Med 1982;307:1476–80.
4. Oberbaum M, Yaniv I, Ben-Gal Y, et al. A randomized, controlled clinical trial of the homeopathic medication Traumeel S in the treatment of chemotherapy-induced stomatitis in children undergoing stem cell transplantation. Cancer 2001;92:684–90.
5. Syrjala KL, Cummings C, Donaldson GW. Hypnosis or cognitive behavioral training for the reduction of pain and nausea during cancer treatment: a controlled clinical trial. Pain 1992;48:137–46.

18

Complementary Therapies for Endocrine Symptoms

This chapter discusses complementary therapies for hot flashes and sexual dysfunction.

HOT FLASHES

Hot flashes are a widely recognized side effect of treatment for hormone-dependent cancers. Approximately two-thirds of breast cancer patients report hot flashes. Of these, 60%, or 40% of all patients, rate their problem as moderately or extremely severe. Hot flashes or sweats are reported by about two-thirds of prostate cancer patients on hormonal treatment and by about one-half of those who undergo orchiectomy. Although symptoms are often said to become less severe with time, no reliable prospective data support this observation.

Hormone replacement therapy, the standard treatment for hot flashes in menopausal women, is not used for patients with breast cancer as it may stimulate the growth of hormone-dependent tumors. A variety of nonhormonal agents show efficacy in randomized trials, including megestrol acetate, clonidine, and selective serotonin reuptake inhibitors such as venlafaxine. However, these drugs are only of modest benefit and are associated with important side effects, including nausea, anorexia, and dry mouth. Many patients turn to integrative therapies in hopes of finding effective relief.

TREATMENT

Several trials of complementary therapies for hot flashes in cancer patients have been conducted. Although most included only patients with breast cancer, their results should be thought of as applicable to those with other hormone-dependent cancers, such as prostate cancer.

Botanicals

The most widely used integrative therapies for hot flashes are botanical agents. Many of these, such as soy and red clover, are purportedly effective on the grounds that they contain estrogen-like substances ("phytoestrogens"). Unfortunately, solid evidence from randomized trials shows that botanicals, in fact, are not effective in providing relief. Studies of hot flashes in menopausal women without cancer failed to find benefit for red clover, flax, Dong Guai, yam, or evening primrose oil. Studies in cancer patients show that both soy and black cohosh are no more effective than placebo for treating hot flashes. Moreover, phytoestrogenic soy products should be avoided by patients with estrogen receptor–positive breast cancer (see Chapter 11).

Vitamin E

Although vitamin E is not traditionally recommended for menopausal symptoms, a clinical trial found that 800 IUs of vitamin E daily reduced hot flashes in breast cancer survivors. Although it did not have a large effect, vitamin E is often recommended because it is inexpensive and relatively safe. Oral vitamin E is well tolerated and safe. High-dosage (>400 IU/daily) should not be taken for long periods of time or by people with coronary heart disease.

Acupuncture

Acupuncture is a popular treatment for hot flashes, and several case series show positive results. For example, in one study of 22 breast cancer patients receiving 8 to 14 acupuncture treatments, the mean number of hot flashes was reduced from 20 to less than two per day, an improvement maintained at a 1-month follow-up. Several randomized trials of acupuncture for hot flashes are underway; clinical recommendations await publication of these results.

Mind–Body Techniques

Vasodilation has a psychological component (blushing is a common example), and several publications describe mind–body techniques used to treat hot flashes. Single-arm studies of hypnosis and relaxation therapy report encouraging results. However, as in the case of acupuncture, no randomized trials are yet published.

SEXUAL DYSFUNCTION

Treatment for cancer can lead to sexual difficulties in a number of ways. Common problems include erectile dysfunction following prostatectomy or radiation therapy, pain, and burning following surgery for gynecologic tumors, and loss of potency, pain, and other difficulties following hormone treatment of breast and prostate cancers. Sexual dysfunction also may result from cytotoxic damage to hormone-producing glands, changes in body image after surgery, and mood disturbance associated with the extreme stress of cancer diagnosis. Counseling, medication such as Viagra, and aids such as lubricants represent the basis of supportive care for cancer patients with sexual dysfunction. Preliminary data suggest that several integrative approaches can help sexual dysfunction.

TREATMENT

Herbs

One of the best-known products for men, Korean red ginseng, was studied in two randomized trials. In one, 45 patients with erectile dysfunction reported an improvement of about one-third in sexual function scores following 900 mg of Korean red ginseng. There was little improvement in control subjects, and the difference between treatments was statistically significant. Conversely, trials of *Gingko biloba* have not supported its effectiveness for this problem.

Randomized trials also support the efficacy of several botanicals for increasing sexual desire, including oral maca for men and both ArginMax, a supplement containing ginseng and ginkgo and Zestra, a topical botanical product, for women. Note that particular care is required in using botanical products promoted for sexual dysfunction, as contamination with prescription drugs appears to be particularly common.

Generally speaking, reported effects have been shown to be independent of hormonal mechanisms. In the trial of Korean red ginseng, for example, there was no difference in testosterone levels between groups; in the maca study, treatment effects were unchanged by statistical adjustment for changes in levels of testosterone and estradiol. These products therefore appear to be safe in patients with hor-

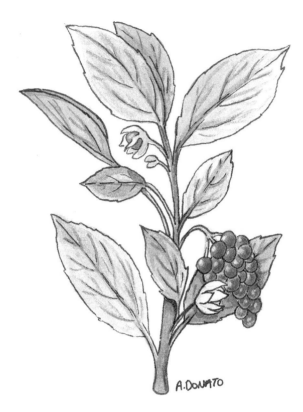

Figure 18-1 Korean red ginseng improves sexual function in men with erectile dysfunction.

mone-dependent cancers. Whether they are effective in such patients, however, has not been studied.

The physiologic and psychologic causes of sexual dysfunction in cancer patients are very different from those in patients without cancer. For example, erectile dysfunction following prostatectomy differs from the nonorganic erectile dysfunction studied in the trials noted above; indeed, in most studies, prostatectomy was an explicit exclusion criterion.

Hypnosis

Preliminary data from randomized trials suggest that hypnosis (see Chapter 7) can improve sexual function in men with nonorganic sexual dysfunction. It does seem reasonable that mind–body complementary therapies may help patients for whom anxiety or depression is a contributing factor in sexual dysfunction (see Chapter 16). Many therapies have been shown to decrease anxiety, improve depression, and improve patients' general sense of well-being.

READINGS AND RESOURCES

1. Barton DL, Loprinzi CL, Quella SK, et al. Prospective evaluation of vitamin E for hot flashes in breast cancer survivors. J Clin Oncol 1998;16:495–500.
2. Hong B, Ji YH, Hong JH, et al. A double-blind crossover study evaluating the efficacy of Korean red ginseng in patients with erectile dysfunction: a preliminary report. J Urol 2002;168:2070–3.
3. Quella SK, Loprinzi CL, Barton DL, et al. Evaluation of soy phytoestrogens for the treatment of hot flashes in breast cancer survivors: A North Central Cancer Treatment Group Trial. J Clin Oncol 2000;18:1068–74.

19

Alternative and Questionable Therapies

Unlike all other chapters in this manual, which review useful complementary therapies, this concluding entry addresses "alternative" therapies, those that typically are promoted for use as literal alternatives to surgery, chemotherapy, radiotherapy, and other mainstream oncologic treatments. Alternative therapies often are invasive, biologically active, and potentially harmful. They may harm directly, through biologic activity, or indirectly, when patients postpone conventional treatment to try them first. This chapter summarizes a dozen of the numerous, currently popular alternative approaches. Given in alphabetical order, these are antineoplastons, Cancell, coral calcium, electrical therapies, energy therapies, Essiac, high-dose vitamins, Laetrile, metabolic therapies, oxygen and ozone therapies, 714X, and shark cartilage.

ANTINEOPLASTON TREATMENT

Antineoplastons were produced by Stanislaw Burzynski in his Houston, Texas clinic. This therapy is promoted especially for pediatric brain tumor patients. Research has not documented the effectiveness of phenylacetate, a metabolite of the amino acid phenylalanine, which makes up 80% of antineoplastons.

CANCELL

Cancell and related products contain a variety of ingredients including catechol, nitric acid, sodium sulfite, potassium hydroxide, sulfuric acid, crocinic acid, and various minerals and vitamins. Proponents claim that their products balance the vibrational frequency of cancer cells and return them to their healthy state. There is no published research evaluating the benefits of Cancell.

CORAL CALCIUM

Coral calcium, derived from the natural matrix of corals, is promoted as a natural calcium supplement to cure cancer. However, none of the purported anticancer benefits are documented. The U.S. Federal Trade Commission (FTC) and Food and Drug Administration (FDA) have issued warnings to numerous Web site operators who tout unsubstantiated benefits for coral calcium.

ELECTRICAL THERAPIES

Electrical therapies include electrodermal testing, bioresonance therapy, biophysical information therapy (BIT), bioenergetic therapy, energy medicine and vibrational medicine. Brand names of devices include Dermatron, Accupath 1000, Vega, Interro, Hubbard E-Meter, Electro-Acuscope 80, and Qigong Machine. Electrical therapies are used to diagnose and treat cancer, allergies, arthritis, and various other chronic diseases. They are based on the idea that electromagnetic oscillations emitted by diseased organs and cancer cells vary from those of healthy cells and can be detected by an electrical galvanic device that measures electrical resistance on the skin, usually along acupuncture points or meridians. Patients are treated with a "radiofrequency electrical signal" said to normalize electrical conductance, strengthen the body's natural oscillations, cancel pathological oscillations via destructive wave interference, and normalize cell metabolism. No evidence supports any of these claims. The FTC recently closed a popular Internet site selling this therapy.

ENERGY THERAPIES

There are numerous types; most involve manipulation of a putative human energy field or use of a "healer's" special gift for energy healing, harkening back to ancient concepts of restoring health (see Chapter 2). Healing of this type, which has remained popular over the centuries primarily in less developed areas of the world, has gained increasing public interest and acceptance in North America and elsewhere. Many healers claim the ability to cure people of cancer. Many patients are convinced of these healers' abilities and decline even to have tumors removed surgically.

ESSIAC

Generally consumed as a tea, this product contains four botanicals: cut or dried burdock root, powdered sheep sorrel root, powdered slippery elm bark, and powdered rhubarb root. Promoters claim that Essiac boosts the immune system, acts as a tonic, and treats cancer and human immunodeficiency virus (HIV). There are no data and no published clinical trials that support claims made for this product. Possible adverse effects include nausea, vomiting, diarrhea, constipation, hypoglycemia, and renal and hepatic toxicity with chronic consumption. Case reports indicate that burdock root contaminated with belladonna has caused atropine-like toxicity.

HIGH-DOSE VITAMINS

High-quality controlled research on the potential benefit of high-dose vitamin C shows no benefit. Moreover, high concentrations of vitamin C may be harmful, as cancer cells selectively uptake vitamin C, suggesting that high doses may feed cancer cells preferentially and can suppress drug-induced cancer cell death. It also may cause other serious problems, such as kidney failure.

LAETRILE

A naturally occurring cyanogenic glycoside derived from nuts, plants, and the pits of certain fruits, primarily apricots, research demonstrates only toxicity and the absence of beneficial effect. Laetrile (amygdalin) is metabolized by beta-glucosidase to cyanide, benzaldehyde, and prunasin. It is illegal in the United States, but is available in Tijuana clinics and on the Internet. It is also known as apricot pits, vitamin B_{17}, mandelonitrile-beta-glucuronide (semisynthetic), mandelonitrile beta-D-gentiobioside (natural product), and prunasin.

METABOLIC THERAPIES

These strict dietary and detoxification regimens sold to prevent and treat cancer and other degenerative diseases are available primarily in Mexican border clinics. Coffee enemas and other aspects of detoxification are based on the early idea that cancer and other diseases are caused by an accumulation of toxic substances in the body (see Chapter 2). Advocates claim that a restrictive diet and detoxification will allow the body to heal naturally.

Therapies such as the Gerson, Kelley, Contreras, Manner, and Gonzalez regimens share this ideology but differ in modality. Diet may be supplemented with digestive enzymes, glandular extracts, megadose vitamins, minerals, or herbal products. Agents such as Bacillus Calmette-Guérin (BCG), gamma globulins, interleukins, hydrazine sulphate, hydrogen peroxide, glandular extracts, or laetrile also may be administered. The strict diets can cause nutritional deficiencies, and some entail potentially toxic doses of supplements or agents. Excessive use of coffee enemas can cause sepsis, dangerous electrolyte deficiencies, and death. Retrospective reviews of the Gerson, Kelley, and Contreras metabolic therapies show no evidence of efficacy.

OXYGEN THERAPIES

Promoters claim that cancer cells grow only in the absence of oxygen, and that introducing oxygen will reverse the cancerous process by suffocating the cell with excess oxygen. However, oxygen neither prevents nor inhibits cancer growth, but rather encourages their growth. Cancer cells grow rapidly in tissues well supplied with oxygen. Claims that adding oxygen to the body creates an oxygen-rich condition in which cancer cells cannot survive sound logical to many patients, rendering oxygen therapies quite popular. This disproved claim stems from long-discredited ideas set forth in the 1930s by Otto Warburg.

714X

Gaston Naessens of Quebec, Canada, developed a dark-field microscope that he terms a "Somatoscope." He claims to examine live blood cells at a magnification of up to 30,000 to see tiny creatures he calls "somatids," which he says are responsible for cancer. Scientists who looked through the dark-field microscope reported that particles seen there are well known by hematologists to be products of red-cell disintegration. Naessens then developed a cancer treatment, 714X (for the 7th and 14th letters in the alphabet—his initials—and "X" for the 24th letter in the alphabet, his year of birth—1924), claiming that 714X can cure cancer, multiple sclerosis, fibromyalgia, and other "degenerative diseases." No clinical trial has been reported, and no evidence supports the existence of somatids or the effectiveness of 714X.

SHARK CARTILAGE

Obtained from the spiny dogfish shark and hammerhead shark, many products contain primarily binding agents or fillers with little or no activity. The FTC has barred manufacturers from making unsubstantiated claims of efficacy for their shark cartilage products. Shark cartilage extracts show antiangiogenic and antitumor activity in vitro and in animal models, but clinical use remains controversial due to unsatisfactory patient outcomes in phase I and II trials in cancer patients. Other research is underway. The U.S. National Cancer Institute Web site (http://cancer.gov) concludes that "bovine (cow) cartilage and shark cartilage have been studied as treatments for cancer and other medical conditions for more than 30 years. The results of human trials are inconclusive." Currently available supplements have no value.

CONCLUSION

It is important for oncology professionals to differentiate between useful complementary therapies that help manage symptoms and alternative therapies promoted for use in place of mainstream cancer care. Most "alternative" cancer cures have not been subjected to clinical trials; the few that have been tested were found ineffective, and promotional claims draw cancer patients to these useless and often expensive bogus therapies.

READINGS AND RESOURCES

1. American Cancer Society. http://www.cancer.org (accessed March 12, 2005).
2. Moertel CG. High-dose vitamin C versus placebo in the treatment of patients with advanced cancer who have had no prior chemotherapy. A randomized double-blind comparison. N Engl J Med 1985;312:137–41.
3. Quackwatch. http://www.quackwatch.org (accessed March 12, 2005).
4. National Institute of Health. http://www.nccam.nih.gov (accessed March 12, 2005).

Index

A

Acupuncture, 12, 73–81, 74f
  adverse effects of, 79
  auricular, 78–79
  in cancer care
    indication for, 78–79
  chemotherapy-induced nausea and
    vomiting, 99–100
  clinical assessment, 76–77
  complications, 139
  for fatigue, 153
  for hot flashes, 168
  mechanisms of action, 75–76
  for mood disturbance, 149
  for nausea and vomiting, 159–161
  needles, 77–78, 77f
    increasing stimulation of, 78–79
  for pain, 138–139
  for prostate cancer, 131
  with serotonin receptor
    antagonists, 100
  smoking cessation, 115
  treatment plan, 76–77
  for xerostomia, 163
AICR. See American Institute for
  Cancer Research (AICR)
ALA. See Alpha linolenic acid
  (ALA)
Alpha linolenic acid (ALA), 54, 54f,
  58, 118
  for pain, 143
Alpha-Tocopheral Beta-Carotene
  (ATBC) Cancer Prevention
  Trial, 116, 125
Alprazolam
  for mood disturbance, 148
American Cancer Society, 44
American Dietetic Association, 43
American ginseng (Panax
  quinquefolius)
  for fatigue, 154
American Institute for Cancer
  Research (AICR), 42
Amygdala
  smoking, 116
Amygdalin, 23t
Androgen
  prostate cancer, 131
Anthracycline, 55

  cardiotoxicity, 100–102
Antibiotics, 45
Anticoagulants, 40
Antineoplaston treatment, 172
Antioxidants, 54–56
Antioxidant supplements
  breast cancer, 99
Antiplatelets, 40
Anxiety, 145, 151–156
  music therapy for, 88f
Apiole
  hepatotoxicity of, 38
Apples, 44
Aristolochia fangchi, 37
Aristolochia manshuriensis, 37
Aromatherapy, 89–90
Arsenic, 36
Artemisia, 22, 24t
Art therapy, 88–89
Asian countries
  breast cancer, 98
Asian ginseng (Panax ginseng)
  for fatigue, 154
Asthma
  essential oils, 89
Astragalus, 23t, 40f
ATBC. See Alpha-Tocopheral Beta-
  Carotene (ATBC) Cancer
  Prevention Trial
Auricular acupuncture, 78–79
Ayurveda, 8–11, 9f
  benefits, 10–11
  cautions, 10–11
  treatment, 10

B

Bacillus Calmette-Guerin (BCG),
  175
Benzodiazepine (alprazolam)
  for mood disturbance, 148
Berberine, 22
Beta-carotene, 54, 58
Beta-Carotene and Retinol Efficacy
  Trial (CARET), 116
Bioenergetic therapy, 173
Biofeedback, 70–71
  for bowel incontinence, 113
  for pain, 141

for prostate cancer, 131
Biophysical information therapy
    (BIT), 173
Bioresonance therapy, 173
Black cohosh
    marker compound for, 34t
Blood pressure
    laughing, 91
Body-based interventions
    for pain, 139
Bodywork, 82–86
Borage
    hepatotoxicity of, 38
Boswellia serrata
    for pain, 141
Botanicals, 17–32
    analysis, 33–35
    anticancer properties of, 23t–32t
    for cancer
        research on, 20–32
    carcinogenicity, 39
    cardiotoxicity, 38
    collection and processing, 20–21
    contaminants, 34–41
    hepatotoxicity, 38
    herb-drug interactions, 33–41, 39
    marker compounds for, 34t
    nephrotoxicities, 37–38
    neurotoxicity, 38
    nomenclature, 19t
    phototoxicity, 38
    regulation, 33–35
    standardization, 33–35
    toxicities, 37
Bowel incontinence, 113
    biofeedback, 113
Brazil nuts
    selenium in, 126
Breast
    lymphatic drainage of, 96f
Breast cancer, 95–105
    dairy products, 97
    diet, 96–97
    herbal products after treatment,
        103–104
    herbal products during treatment,
        99–103
    prevention of, 96–99
    soy products, 98–99, 98f
Brown tonic, 49

C
Cachexia, 165
    pancreatic cancer, 113

Calcium
    colon cancer, 107
    coral, 173
Calories
    breast cancer, 96
CAM. *See* Complementary and
    alternative medicine (CAM)
Cancell, 172–173
Cancer
    antioxidant supplements for, 55
    biofeedback for, 71
    botanicals, 17–18
    dance therapy, 90
    herbals for, 22
    vegetarianism risk for, 49
Cancer pain, 135–144
Capillary electrophoresis (CE), 33
Capsaicin
    for pain, 140
CARET. *See* Beta-Carotene and
    Retinol Efficacy Trial (CARET)
Carnitine, 101
Cat's claw
    marker compound for, 34t
Cayenne
    marker compound for, 34t
CB. *See* Compression bandaging
    (CB)
CE. *See* Capillary electrophoresis
    (CE)
Chamomile extract, 108
Chaparral
    hepatotoxicity of, 38
Chemotherapy-induced nausea and
    vomiting
    acupuncture, 99–100
    acupuncture for, 12
    antioxidant supplements for, 55
    breast cancer, 99–100
Children
    hypnosis, 67
    leukemia
        art therapy for, 89
Chinese herbs
    for pain, 141
Chinese immigrants
    pelvic cancer, 124
Chinese licorice, 130
Chiropractic manipulations
    for pain, 140
Chondroitin
    for pain, 140
Chronic pain
    acupuncture for, 12, 80

Chrysanthemum, 130
Cingulate cortex
  smoking, 116
Cinnamon bark, 19t
Cisplatin, 118
Clover
  marker compound for, 34t
Coenzyme Q10, 55f, 101
Coffee enemas, 50, 175
Cognitive meditation
  for nausea and vomiting, 159
Colorectal cancer, 107
  polysaccharide K, 110
Coltsfoot
  hepatotoxicity of, 38
Comfrey
  hepatotoxicity of, 38
Complementary and alternative
    medicine (CAM), 3–4, 123
  adverse effects, 6
  breast cancer, 95
  evolving terminology of, 4–6
  prevalence of, 3–4
Complications, 54
Compression bandaging (CB),
    104–105
Constipation, 161–162
ConsumerLabs, 53
Contreras, 175
Cooked foods, 46t
Coral calcium, 173
Coriolus versicolor, 24t, 110–111,
    110f
Corydalis yanhusuo
  for pain, 141
Crotalaria, 38
Cyclooxygenase-2 (COX-2)
    inhibitors
  colon cancer, 107
Cytochrome P-450 (CYP) 3A4, 39,
    109, 149

D
Daidzein
  pelvic cancer, 124
Damiana *(Turnera diffusa),* 112
Dance therapy, 90
DDT. *See*
    Dichlorodiphenyltrichloroethane
    (DDT)
Depression, 145, 151–156
  music therapy for, 88f
Dexrazoxane, 56
Diabetes, 119

Diarrhea, 161–162
Dichlorodiphenyltrichloroethane
    (DDT), 35–36
Diet, 15, 42–51
  low-fat
    colon cancer, 107
  Mediterranean, 48
  for pain, 143
Dietary cancer treatments, 47–48
Dietary recommendations, 42–43
Dietary Supplement Health and
    Education Act (DSHEA), 35,
    52–53, 53
Dietary supplements, 6, 52–63
  for pain, 140
Digestive enzymes, 45–46
D-limonene, 24t, 58–59
Doctrine of Signatures, 19
Dong guai, 25t
Doshas, 9
Doxorubicin, 108
DSHEA. *See* Dietary Supplement
    Health and Education Act
    (DSHEA)
Dumping syndrome, 112
Dyer's woad, 130
Dyspnea
  lung cancer, 120

E
Ear seeds
  acupuncture, 78
Earth, 12t
Echinacea, 17
  hepatotoxicity of, 38
  marker compound for, 34t
EFA. *See* Essential fatty acids (EFA)
Eicosapentaenoic acid (EPA), 113
Electrical therapy, 173
Electroacupuncture, 100
Electrodermal testing, 173
Element correspondences, 12t
Eleutherococcus senticosus
  for fatigue, 154
Ellagic acid, 25t
Endocrine symptoms, 167–176
End-of-life care
  mind-body therapies, 71
Endorphins, 66
  laughing, 91
Energy medicine, 173–174
  for pain, 142

EORTC. *See* European
    Organization for Research and
    Treatment of Cancer (EORTC)
EPA. *See* Eicosapentaenoic acid
    (EPA)
Esophagectomy, 112
Essential fatty acids (EFA)
    for pain, 143
Essential oils, 20, 89–90
    allergic reaction to, 89
Essiac, 25t, 174
Estrogen
    prostate cancer, 131
Etoposide, 108
European Organization for
    Research and Treatment of
    Cancer (EORTC), 119
EUROSCAN, 122
Exercise, 82–83
    reducing cancer risk, 83

F
Fatigue, 82–83, 151–152
    acupuncture, 153
    dietary supplements, 154–155
Fats
    breast cancer, 96
FDA. *See* US Food and Drug
    Administration (FDA)
Feverfew
    marker compound for, 34t
Fiber
    colon cancer, 107
Fibrosis, 116
Fire, 12t
Fish oil
    for pain, 143
5-fluorouracil (5-FU), 57
    causing mucositis, 108–109
5-hydroxytryptamine (5-HT$_3$), 157
Flavonols, 116
Flaxseed, 59
fMRI. *See* Functional magnetic
    resonance imaging (fMRI)
Folate
    colon cancer, 107
Folic acid, 59
    for fatigue, 154
Food Guide Pyramid, 43
Foot massage
    for mood disturbance, 147
Fruits
    colon cancer, 107
    lycopene, 127

5-FU. *See* 5-fluorouracil (5-FU)
Functional magnetic resonance
    imaging (fMRI), 138
    acupuncture, 76

G
GABA. *See* Gamma-aminobutyric
    acid (GABA)
Gamma-aminobutyric acid (GABA),
    138
    for mood disturbances, 150
GAP. *See* Good agricultural practice
    (GAP) farms
Garlic, 17
    marker compound for, 34t
Gas chromatography (GC), 33
Gastrectomy, 112
Gastric motility, 112
Gastrointestinal cancer, 106–113
    diet, 107
    dietary supplements, 107–108
    herbal products after treatment,
        111–113
    herbal products during treatment,
        108–111
    postoperative recovery, 111
    prevention of, 107–108, 107f
    wound healing, 111
Gastrointestinal symptoms,
    157–165
GC. *See* Gas chromatography (GC)
Genistein
    pelvic cancer, 124
Gerson, 175
Gerson, Max, 49–50
Gerson Institute, 50
Gerson regimen, 49–50
Ginger root, 19t, 162
Gingko extract, 118
Ginkgo biloba, 17, 35
    marker compound for, 34t
    for sexual dysfunction, 169
Ginkgo flavone glycosides, 35
Ginkgo leaf, 19t
Ginseng, 17, 26t, 155f
    for fatigue, 154
    Korean red, 170f
        for sexual dysfunction, 169
    marker compound for, 34t
Glucans, 102–103
Glucosamine
    for pain, 140
Glutathione, 118
Glycyrrhiza glabra (licorice), 99

Goldenseal
    marker compound for, 34t
Gonzalez, 175
Good agricultural practice (GAP)
    farms, 20
Government, 6
Grapefruit
    lycopene, 126–127
Grapefruit juice
    cytochrome P-450 (CYP) 3A4,
        110
Grape skin extract
    marker compound for, 34t
Graviola, 26t
Green bell peppers, 44
Green tea, 27t
    marker compound for, 34t
Growth hormone, 45
Guarana (Paullinia cupana), 112
Guava
    lycopene, 126–127
Guided imagery, 68–69

H
Han dynasty, 11
Hawthorn
    marker compound for, 34t
Hawthorn berry, 19t
Healing touch
    for pain, 142
Health Professionals Follow-Up
    Study (HPFS), 126
Heavy metals, 36
Heliotropium, 38
Herbalism, 18
Herbal medicine
    in China, 17
    for mood disturbance, 149–150
    for nausea and vomiting, 161
    for pain, 141
Herbology, 18
Herbs, 17–32
    hepatotoxicity, 13
Herceptin, 102–103
High-dose vitamins, 174
High-performance liquid
    chromatography (HPLC), 33
Hippocampus
    smoking, 116
HIV. See Human immunodeficiency
    virus (HIV)
Homeopathy, 13–14
    benefits, 14
    cautions, 14

treatment, 14
Honeysuckle flower, 19t
Hops, 99
Hormone replacement therapy, 167
Hot flashes, 167
    acupuncture, 168
    breast cancer, 104
Hoxsey, Harry, 49
Hoxsey therapy, 49
HPFS. See Health Professionals
    Follow-Up Study (HPFS)
HPLC. See High-performance liquid
    chromatography (HPLC)
5-HT$_3$. See 5-hydroxytryptamine (5-
    HT$_3$)
Huang Lian, 22, 22f, 27t, 162
Human immunodeficiency virus
    (HIV), 119, 138, 174
Human root, 19
Humor therapy, 90–91
Humulus lupus (hops), 99
Hydrazine sulfate, 119
5-hydroxytryptamine (5-HT$_3$), 157
Hyperglycemia
    postprandial, 112
Hypnosis, 66–68
    children, 67
    contraindications for, 68
    for pain, 142
    for sexual dysfunction, 170–171
    smoking cessation, 115
Hypnotherapy, 111
Hypnotic state, 67

I
ICAM-1. See Intercellular adhesion
    molecule (ICAM-1)
Ifosfamide, 108
IGF. See Insulin-like growth factors
    (IGF)
Immune-enhancing botanicals, 41
Indirubin, 22, 28t
Indole-3-carbinol, 28t
Information therapy
    biophysical, 173
Insulin-like growth factors (IGF), 45
Integrative medicine, 5
Integrative oncology, 3–7
Intercellular adhesion molecule
    (ICAM-1), 63
International Association for the
    Study of Pain, 136
Intradermal needles
    acupuncture, 77–78

Irinotecan
  drug-herb interaction, 109–110
Isoflavones, 57

J
Japanese immigrants
  pelvic cancer, 124
Juicing, 46–47
Juzen-taiho-to, 22

K
Kampo botanical medicine, 162
Kapha, 9
Kava
  for mood disturbances, 149, 150
Kava kava
  marker compound for, 34t
Kelley, 175
Korean red ginseng, 170f
  for sexual dysfunction, 169

L
Lactovegetarians, 48
Laetrile, 49–50, 174
Laughing
  blood pressure, 91
L-carnitine, 101
Lead, 36
Lead poisoning
  with ayurveda, 10
Lentinan, 28t–29t
Leukemia
  children
    art therapy for, 89
Licorice, 99, 162
  marker compound for, 34t
Lifestyle, 15
Limonene, 24t, 58–59
Liver cirrhosis, 108
Livingston-Wheeler therapy, 50
Low-fat diet
  colon cancer, 107
Lung cancer, 115–127
  diet, 116–117
  dietary supplements, 116–117
  herbal products after treatment,
    121–122
  herbal products during treatment,
    116–120
  postthoracotomy pain, 121
  prevention of, 115–117
    second primary tumor, 121–122
  quality of life, 119–120
Lutein, 54

Lycopene, 54, 60, 126–127
Lymphedema
  breast cancer, 104

M
Macrobiotics
  for cancer, 47–48
Maitake, 22f, 29t
Manipulative interventions
  for pain, 139
Manner, 175
Manual lymphatic drainage (MLD),
  104
Massage therapy, 85
  for fatigue, 152, 155–156
  for mood disturbance, 146–147
  for nausea and vomiting, 158
  for pain, 139–140
  types of, 85–86
Mass spectrometry (MS), 33
MBSR. *See* Mindfulness-based stress
  reduction (MBSR)
Meditation, 69–71
  cognitive
    for nausea and vomiting, 159
  physiologic change, 70
Mediterranean diet, 48
Melatonin, 54, 60
Melzack's gate theory, 136
Mercury, 36
Metabolic dietary regimens, 49–50
Metabolic therapies, 175
Metal, 12t
Methotrexate, 108
Methylsulfonylmethane (MSM)
  for pain, 140
Milk thistle
  marker compound for, 34t
Mind-body therapies, 65–71
  for end-of-life care, 71
  for fatigue, 153–154, 155–156
  for hot flashes, 168
  for mood disturbance, 147–148
  for nausea and vomiting, 159
  for oral mucositis, 165
  for pain, 141
  prostate cancer, 131
Mindfulness-based stress reduction
  (MBSR), 69, 84–85
Mistletoe, 29t
Mistletoe extract, 119
MLD. *See* Manual lymphatic
  drainage (MLD)
Mood disturbance, 145–151

acupuncture, 149
integrative therapy for, 151
Movement therapy
for pain, 142
MS. *See* Mass spectrometry (MS)
MSM. *See* Methylsulfonylmethane
(MSM)
Mung bean, 19t
Music therapy, 87–88, 88f
for fatigue, 152–153
for mood disturbance, 148–149

N
N-acetylcysteine, 54, 60–61
National Comprehensive Cancer
Network (NCCN), 153
Naturopathic doctors (ND), 15
Naturopathic treatments, 15t
Naturopathy, 14–16
benefits, 15–16
cautions, 15–16
treatment, 15
Nausea and vomiting, 157–158. *See
also* Chemotherapy-induced
nausea and vomiting
acupuncture, 78–79, 159–161
cognitive meditation, 159
NCCN. *See* National
Comprehensive Cancer
Network (NCCN)
ND. *See* Naturopathic doctors (ND)
Needling sensation, 78
Nerium oleander, 23t
Neuropathy
acupuncture, 80–81
Noni, 30t
Non-small cell lung cancer
(NSCLC), 118, 119
Nonsteroidal anti-inflammatory
drugs (NSAID), 136
colon cancer, 107
North American market, 6
Nurses' Health Study, 107
Nutrition, 15, 42–51
Nutritional Prevention of Skin
Cancer trial, 125

O
Ohsawa, George, 47
Olive oil
lycopene, 127
Omega-3 fatty acids
for pain, 143
Oral mucositis, 164–165

Organic foods, 43–44
Osteoporosis
breast cancer, 103–104
Ovarian cancer
herbs, 18
Ovolactovegetarians, 48
Oxygen therapies, 175

P
Paclitaxel
neuropathy, 102
Pain
acupuncture, 138–139
alpha linolenic acid for, 143
with anxiety, 67
biofeedback, 141
Boswellia serrata, 141
cancer, 135–144
capsaicin, 140
Chinese herbs, 141
chronic
acupuncture for, 12, 80
hypnosis for, 66
integrative management approach,
137–138
pancreatic cancer, 113
Palliative care
in cancer patients
essential oils, 89
Panax ginseng, 19
for fatigue, 154
Panax quinquefolius
for fatigue, 154
Pancreatic cancer cachexia, 113
Pancreatic cancer pain, 113
Pancreatin, 45
Pau d'Arco, 30t
Paullinia cupana, 112
PC SPES, 22, 30t, 36f, 37, 130
Peaches, 44
Pelvic cancer
Chinese immigrants, 124
diet, 124
prevention of, 124–126
selenium, 125–126
soy, 124
vitamin E, 124–125
Pelvic muscle exercise (PME), 131
Pelvis
anatomy of, 123f
Peppermint
marker compound for, 34t
Pesticides, 43–44, 44
P-glycoprotein, 40

Pharmacognosy, 18
Physicians' Health Study, 107
Phytoestrogens, 41, 57
  for hot flashes, 168
  soy, 99
Phytomedicinals, 18
Pitta, 9
Plants
  classification of, 18–19
Platinum compounds, 55
Platinum-induced neuropathy,
  118–119
PME. *See* Pelvic muscle exercise
  (PME)
Pneumonitis, 116
Pneumothorax, 139
Polysaccharide K (PSK), 110–111
Polysaccharide P (PSP), 110–111
Postprandial hyperglycemia, 112
Prakruti, 9
Prana, 10
Progenitor cryptocides, 50
Prostate cancer, 48, 57, 123–132
  acupuncture, 131
  biofeedback, 131
  herbals after treatment, 130–132
  herbals during treatment,
    127–130
  lycopene, 128, 129f
  osteoporosis, 131–132
  PC SPES for, 37, 129–130
  pelvic symptoms, 130–131
  polysaccharides, 128–129
  selenium, 128
  sexual dysfunction, 131
  soy, 127–128
  vasomotor symptoms, 131
Prostate-specific antigen (PSA), 127
PSA. *See* Prostate-specific antigen
  (PSA)
Pseudoginseng, 130
PSK. *See* Polysaccharide K (PSK)
PSP. *See* Polysaccharide P (PSP)
Psychostimulants
  for fatigue, 155
Pyrrolizidine alkaloids
  hepatotoxicity of, 38

Q
Qi, 10, 12
Qigong, 12, 84
Quercetin, 54, 61
Questionable therapies, 172–176

R
Rabdosia, 130
Radiation dermatitis, 103
Radiation therapy, 55, 116
  for prostate cancer, 83
Raw foods, 46t
Recombinant bovine growth
    hormone (rBGH), 45
Red clover, 99
Red ginseng
  Korean, 170f
    for sexual dysfunction, 169
Reiki
  for pain, 142
Reishi mushroom, 130
Relaxation techniques, 65
ReliefBand, 160
Ren Shen, 19, 19t
Rose hip
  lycopene, 126–127
  marker compound for, 34t

S
S-adenosyl-L-methionine (SAMe)
  for pain, 140
Saw palmetto, 130
  marker compound for, 34t
Selective estrogen receptor
    modulators (SERMS)
  breast cancer, 98
  pelvic cancer, 124
Selective serotonin reuptake
    inhibitors (SSRI)
  for mood disturbance, 149
Selenium, 54, 61–62
  foods rich in, 126t
Selenium and Vitamin E Cancer
    Prevention Trial (SELECT), 57,
    61–62, 125, 126
Selenium supplements, 105
Self-hypnosis
  for pain, 138
Senecio, 38
Senna
  marker compound for, 34t
Senses, 87–91
Sequential pneumatic compression
    (SPC), 104
Serotonin receptor antagonists
  acupuncture, 100
714X, 175–176
Sexual dysfunction, 169
Shark cartilage, 176
Shi-quan-da-bu-tang, 22

Sho-saiko-to, 22
Siberian ginseng *(Eleutherococcus senticosus)*
  for fatigue, 154
Singapore General Hospital, 90
Skullcap, 130, 162
Smoking cessation
  acupuncture, 115
  lung cancer, 115–116
Soy, 31t, 57
  marker compound for, 34t
SPC. *See* Sequential pneumatic compression (SPC)
SSRI. *See* Selective serotonin reuptake inhibitors (SSRI)
St. John's wort, 39, 109f
  marker compound for, 34t
  for mood disturbances, 149, 150f
Stephania tetrandra, 37
Sun soup, 31t

T
Tai chi, 12, 83–84
TCM. *See* Traditional Chinese Medicine (TCM)
Tea, 174
TENS. *See* Transcutaneous electrical nerve stimulation (TENS)
Tetrahydrocannabinol (THC), 20
Therapeutic nutrition, 15t
Thin-layer chromatography (TLC), 33
Tibetan yoga, 84, 153
TJ-9, 108
TJ-14, 162
TLC. *See* Thin-layer chromatography (TLC)
Tocopherol
  pelvic cancer, 124
Tocotrienol
  pelvic cancer, 124
Tomatoes, 44, 48
  lycopene, 126–127
Traditional Chinese Medicine (TCM), 11–12, 47, 83
  benefits, 13
  cautions, 13
  treatment, 12–13
Trance, 67
Transcendental meditation, 11
Transcutaneous electrical nerve stimulation (TENS), 120
  lung cancer, 121
Trastuzumab (Herceptin), 102–103

Traumeel S., 164
Trifolium pratense (red clover), 99
Trul khor, 153
Tsa lung, 153
Tuna
  selenium in, 126
Turkey tail, 110
Turmeric, 32t
  for pain, 140
Turnera diffusa, 112

U
Ubiquinone, 62
Ultraviolet-visible (UV-VIS), 33
United States Pharmacopeia Dietary Supplement Verification Program, 53
Urinary incontinence
  biofeedback for, 71
US Food and Drug Administration (FDA), 6, 33, 52–53

V
Valerian
  for mood disturbances, 149–150, 150
Vascular cell adhesion molecule-1 (VCAM-1), 63
Vata, 9
Vegans, 48
Vegetables
  colon cancer, 107
  lycopene, 127
Vegetarianism, 48–49
Vibrational medicine, 173
Virulizin, 111
Visualization, 68–69
Vitamin(s), 52–63
  high-dose, 174
  quality control of, 52–53
  regulation of, 52–53
Vitamin A
  lung cancer, 121–122
Vitamin B12
  for fatigue, 154
Vitamin C, 56f, 62
Vitamin E, 62–63
  for hot flashes, 168
Vomiting. *See* Nausea and vomiting

W
Warfarin, 40
Watchful waiting
  for prostate cancer, 127

Water, 12t
Watermelon
  lycopene, 126–127
Wheeler, Livingston, 51
Wild yam
  marker compound for, 34t
Women's Health Initiative (WHI), 97
Women's Healthy and Lifestyle Study (WHEL), 97
Women's Intervention Nutrition Study (WINS), 97
Wood, 12t
World Cancer Research Fund, 42
World Health Organization
  three-step ladder for cancer pain relief, 137

X
714X, 175–176
Xenoestrogens, 45
Xerostomia, 162–163
  acupuncture, 81
  acupuncture for, 163
Xiao-chai-hu-tang, 22

Y
Yang, 12t, 47
Yellow Emperor's Inner Classic, 11
Yin, 12t, 47
Yoga, 84–85
  for pain, 138
Yun zhi, 110

Z
Zinc, 54